Certified Coding Associate (CCA) Exam Preparation

Dorine L. Bennett, EdD, MBA, RHIA, FAHIMA and
Kathy L. Dorale, RHIA, CCS, CCS-P
Editors

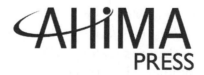

PRESS

ISBN: 978-1-58426-256-5
AHIMA Product No.: AC400310

AHIMA Staff:
Katie Greenock, Editorial and Production Coordinator
Karen M. Kostick, RHIT, CCS, CCS-P, Technical Review
Ashley Sullivan, Assistant Editor
Pamela Woolf, Developmental Editor
Ken Zielske, Director of Publications

American Health Information Management Association
233 North Michigan Avenue, 21st Floor
Chicago, Illinois 60601-5809
ahima.org

Contents

On the CD-ROM

Practice Questions

Practice Exam 1

Practice Exam 2

Practice Exam 3—*Bonus Exam*

References with Links

Printable Blank Answer Sheets

About the Editors

Dorine L. Bennett, EdD, MBA, RHIA, FAHIMA is associate professor and director of the HIM programs at Dakota State University. Prior to joining the faculty at DSU, Dorine worked in the health information management field in settings such as an acute care hospital, a community health office, and a long-term care system as well as independently contracting as a workshop instructor and consultant for long-term care facilities and acute care and specialty hospitals.

Dorine has completed her undergraduate degrees in health information technology (AS) and health information administration (BS) and earned a master of business administration degree with an emphasis in management of information systems (MBA). She recently earned her doctorate degree in educational administration in adult and higher education.

She has served on a number of committees for the American Health Information Management Association and chaired the AHIMA Fellowship Review Committee. Dorine has been president and director of education for the South Dakota Health Information Management Association, as well as leading and serving on a number of committees for the state association. She is also an accreditation site reviewer for the Commission on Accreditation for Health Informatics and Information Management Education (CAHIIM).

Kathy L. Dorale, RHIA, CCS, CCS-P is the vice president of health information management at Avera Health in Sioux Falls, South Dakota. Kathy provides coding and billing reviews and education for Avera Health's 29 hospitals and multifacility healthcare settings in a five-state region. She has experience working with electronic medical records and revenue cycle initiatives collaboratively with Avera Hospitals. Prior to working at Avera's corporate office, Kathy was the director of health information management, business office and registration areas in acute care hospital settings with experience in contract work for long-term care.

Kathy has completed her undergraduate degree in health information administration (BS) and is currently pursuing a masters of science in health informatics at Dakota State University.

She has also served as president and treasurer for the South Dakota Health Information Management Association, as well as serving on several committees for the state association. She enjoys speaking engagements on coding and reimbursement topics to affiliated local and state associations and guest speaking for Dakota State University. She also serves as the vice president on the Provider Roundtable committee with providers across the states. The committee provides comment and testimony on reimbursement and coding issues to the Centers of Medicare and Medicaid-appointed task force during open comment period for the outpatient perspective payment system, biannually, on behalf of all providers.

About the CD-ROM

The CD-ROM accompanying this book contains 200 practice multiple choice questions, three timed, self-scoring practice exams (with 100 questions each) that can be run in practice mode or exam simulation mode, and URL links to some of the references used in this book.

To install the practice exams on your computer:

1. Insert the CD-ROM in your computer's CD/DVD drive.

2. Double-click the .exe file.

3. When asked if you would like to extract files from this archive, select Yes.

4. Accept the license agreement.

5. If offered an installation path, choose the default path suggested.

6. A message will appear stating that the files have been successfully extracted.

7. The Setup Wizard will open.

8. Follow on-screen instructions through setup and install.

Windows Vista users must right-click the .exe file icon and select Run as Administrator. Minimum system requirements: Intel Pentium II 450MHz or faster processor (or equivalent) with 128MB of RAM running Microsoft Windows 2000, XP, Vista, or Windows 7.

The exam simulations are written for a Microsoft Windows environment. To run the test simulations on a Macintosh, you will need to simulate a Windows environment using additional software for a Mac, such as Apple's Bootcamp. AHIMA cannot guarantee this CD will run on a Mac.

This software product is designed to work on Windows 2000, XP, Vista, and Windows 7. Under most circumstances, installation will be easy. To begin the installation, double-click the Program icon. If you have problems with installation, open the "Read me" file on the CD-ROM for help.

Windows Vista users may get an error message on installation. Windows Vista users should right-click the .exe file icon and select Run as Administrator. The program should then extract and install. However, in some controlled environments (such as corporate environments where users are locked down), the process gets a bit more complex. As part of the installation process, some .dll and .ocx files are silently registered into the system registry. This process requires administrative rights, and in some cases, the end user may need to have his or her privileges elevated to install the software. Administrative rights are not needed to actually use the software.

In **Windows Vista**, users without administrative rights will automatically be prompted for the administrative password during the installation. If the user does not have administrative rights, the application, and the shortcut to the application, will not be created on their account—but instead on the administrative user's account. This is obviously not the desired result, but is a consequence of the way Windows Vista works.

About the CCA Exam

The CCA distinguishes coders by exhibiting commitment and demonstrating coding competencies across all settings, including both hospitals and physician practices. Based on job analysis standards and state-of-the art test constuction, the CCA is creating a larger pool of qualified coders ready to meet potential employers' needs. The CCA designation has been nationally accepted standard of achievement in the health information management field since 2002, and is the only HIM credential worldwide currently accredited by the National Commission for Certifying Agencies (NCCA).

Detailed information about the certified coding associate (CCA) exam including academic eligibility requirements, frequently asked questions, and an exam application can be found at ahima.org/certification.

Exam Competency Statements

The multiple choice items on the CCA exam are designed to test three different cognitive abilities: recall, application, and analysis. These levels represent an organized way to identify the performance that practitioners will utilize on the job. An explanation of the three cognitive levels is provided here:

Cognitive Level	Purpose	Performance Required
Recall (RE)	Primarily measures memory	Identify terms, specific facts, methods, procedures, basic concepts, basic theories, principles, and processes.
Application (AP)	Measures simple interpretation of limited data	Apply concepts and principles to new situations; recognize relationships among data; apply laws and theories to practical situations; calculate solutions to mathematical problems; interpret charts and translate graphic data; classify items; interpret information.
Analysis (AN)	Measures the application of knowledge to solving a specific problem and the assembly of various elements into a meaningful whole	Select an appropriate solution for responsive action; revise policy, procedure, or plan; evaluate a solution, case scenario, report, or plan; compare solutions, plans, ideas, or aspects of a problem; evaluate information or a situation; perform multiple calculations to arrive at one answer.

A certification exam is based on an explicit set of competencies. These competencies have been determined through a job analysis study of practitioners. The competencies are subdivided into domains and tasks, as listed here. The exam tests only content pertaining to these competencies. Each domain is allocated a predefined number of questions at specific cognitive levels to make up the exam.

Domain 1: Health Records and Data Content (20%)

- Collect and maintain health data.
- Analyze health records to ensure that documentation supports the patient's diagnosis and procedures, and reflects progress, clinical findings, and discharge status.
- Request patient-specific documentation from other sources (for example, ancillary departments, physicians office, and so on).
- Apply clinical vocabularies and terminologies used in the organization's health information systems.

Domain 2: Health Information Requirements and Standards (14%)

- Evaluate the accuracy and completeness of the patient record as defined by organizational policy and external regulations and standards.
- Monitor compliance with organization-wide health record documentation guidelines.
- Report compliance finding according to organization policy.
- Assist in preparing the organization for accreditation, licensing, and/or certification surveys.

Domain 3: Clinical Classification Systems (36%)

- Use electronic applications to support clinical classification and coding (for example, encoders).
- Assign diagnosis and procedure codes using ICD-9-CM official coding guidelines.
  - Assign principal diagnosis (inpatient) or first listed diagnosis (outpatient).
  - Assign secondary diagnosis(es), including complications and comorbidities (CC).
  - Assign principal and secondary procedure(s).
- Assign procedure codes using CPT coding guidelines.
- Assign appropriate HCPCS codes.
- Identify discrepancies between coded data and supporting documentation.
- Consult reference materials to facilitate code assignment.

Domain 4: Reimbursement Methodologies (10%)

- Validate the data collected for appropriate reimbursement.
  - Validate diagnosis-related groups (DRGs).
  - Validate ambulatory payment classifications (APCs).
- Comply with the National Correct Coding Initiative.
- Verify the national and local coverage determinations (NDC/LDC) for medical necessity.

Domain 5: Information and Communication Technologies (6%)

- Use computer to ensure data collection, storage, analysis, and reporting of information.
- Use common software applications (for example, word processing, spreadsheets, e-mail) in the execution of work processes.
- Use specialized software in the completion of HIM processes.

Domain 6: Privacy, Confidentiality, Legal, and Ethical Issues (14%)

- Apply policies and procedures for access and disclosure of personal health information.
- Release patient-specific data to authorized individuals.
- Apply ethical standards of practice.
- Recognize and report privacy issues/problems.
- Protect data integrity and validity using software or hardware technology.

CCA Exam Specifications

The CCA exam consists of 100 multiple choice questions. Candidates have two hours to complete the exam.

For exams scheduled on or after March 31, 2010, the CCA exam is based on ICD-9-CM codes effective October 1, 2009, and CPT codes effective January 1, 2010. All candidates will have to present the 2010 version of the ICD-9 and CPT codebooks in order to test on or after March 31, 2010. If a candidate presents the incorrect codebooks at the testing center, he or she will be turned away and will forfeit the testing fee. For a complete listing of allowable codebooks, visit ahima.org/certification.

How to Use This Book and CD

The CCA practice questions and practice exams in this book and on the accompanying CD-ROM test knowledge of content pertaining to the CCA competencies published by AHIMA. The 500 multiple choice practice questions and exams in this book and CD-ROM are presented in a similar format to those that might be found on the CCA exam.

This book contains 200 multiple choice practice questions and two multiple choice practice exams (with 100 questions each). Because each question is identified with one of the six CCA domains, you will be able to determine whether you need knowledge or skill building in particular areas of the exam. Most questions provide an answer rationale and reference. Pursuing the sources of these references will help build your knowledge and skills.

To most effectively use this book, work through all of the practice questions first. This will help identify areas in which you may need further preparation. After going through the practice questions, take one of the practice exams. Again, for the questions that you answer incorrectly, refresh your knowledge by reading the associated references. Continue in the same manner with the second and third practice exams. Blank answer sheets are provided on pages 135–37.

The CD-ROM contains the same 200 practice questions and two timed practice exams printed in the book, a third *bonus* practice exam, and references with live links. These timed, self-scoring exams can be run in practice mode—which allows you to work at your own pace—or exam simulation mode—which simulates the two-hour, timed exam experience. You may retake the practice questions and exams as many times as you like. The practice questions and simulated practice exams on CD can be set to be presented in random order, or you may choose to go through the questions in sequential order by domain. You may also choose to practice or test your skills on specific domains. For example, if you would like to build your skills in domain 3, you may choose only domain 3 questions for a given practice session.

Certified Coding Associate
Exam Preparation

Practice Questions

Domain 1: Health Records and Data Content

1. Which of the following elements is **not** a component of most patient records?

    a. Patient identification

    b. Clinical history

    c. Financial information

    d. Test results

2. Which of the following is not a characteristic of high-quality healthcare data?

    a. Data relevancy

    b. Data currency

    c. Data consistency

    d. Data accountability

3. Identify where the following information would be found in the acute care record: Following induction of an adequate general anesthesia, and with the patient supine on the padded table, the left upper extremity was prepped and draped in the standard fashion.

    a. Anesthesia report

    b. Physician progress notes

    c. Operative report

    d. Recovery room record

4. Identify where the following information would be found in the acute care record: "CBC: WBC 12.0, RBC 4.65, HGB 14.8, HCT 43.3, MCV 93."

    a. Medical laboratory report

    b. Pathology report

    c. Physical examination

    d. Physician orders

5. Identify where the following information would be found in the acute care record: "PA and Lateral Chest: The lungs are clear. The heart and mediastinum are normal in size and configuration. There are minor degenerative changes of the lower thoracic spine."

    a. Medical laboratory report

    b. Physical examination

    c. Physician progress note

    d. Radiography report

6. The following is documented in an acute care record: "HEENT: Reveals the tympanic membranes, nares, and pharynx to be clear. No obvious head trauma. CHEST: Good bilateral chest sounds." In which of the following would this documentation appear?

    a. History

    b. Pathology report

    c. Physical examination

    d. Operation report

7. The following is documented in an acute care record: "Microscopic: Sections are of squamous mucosa with no atypia." In which of the following would this documentation appear?

    a. History

    b. Pathology report

    c. Physical examination

    d. Operation report

8. The following is documented in an acute care record: "Admit to 3C. Diet: NPO Meds: Compazine 10mg IV Q 6 PRN." In which of the following would this documentation appear?

    a. Admission order

    b. History

    c. Physical examination

    d. Progress notes

9. The following is documented in an acute care record: "38 weeks gestation, Apgars 8/9, 6# 9.8 oz, good cry." In which of the following would this documentation appear?

    a. Admission note

    b. Clinical laboratory

    c. Newborn record

    d. Physician order

10. The following is documented in an acute care record: "Atrial fibrillation with rapid ventricular response, left axis deviation, left bundle branch block." In which of the following would this documentation appear?

    a. Admission order

    b. Clinical laboratory report

    c. ECG report

    d. Radiology report

11. The following is documented in an acute care record: "I was asked to evaluate this Level I trauma patient with an open left humeral epicondylar fracture. Recommendations: Proceed with urgent surgery for debridement, irrigation, and treatment of open fracture." In which of the following would this documentation appear?

    a. Admission note

    b. Consultation report

    c. Discharge summary

    d. Nursing progress notes

12. The following is documented in an acute care record: "Spoke to the attending re: my assessment. Provided adoption and counseling information. Spoke to CPS re: referral. Case manager to meet with patient and family." In which of the following would this documentation appear?

    a. Admission note

    b. Nursing note

    c. Physician progress note

    d. Social work note

13. A coder notes that the patient is taking prescribed Haldol. The final diagnoses on the progress notes include diabetes mellitus, acute pharyngitis, and malnutrition. What condition might the coder suspect the patient has and should query the physician?

    a. Insomnia

    b. Hypertension

    c. Mental or behavior problems

    d. Rheumatoid arthritis

14. In conducting a qualitative analysis to ensure that documentation in the health record supports the diagnosis of the patient, what documentation would a coder look for to substantiate the diagnosis of aspiration pneumonia?

    a. Diffuse parenchymal lung disease on x-ray

    b. Patient has history of inhaled food, liquid, or oil

    c. Positive culture for Pneumocystis carinii

    d. Positive culture for Streptococcus pneumoniae

15. In conducting a qualitative review the clinical documentation specialist sees that the nursing staff has documented the patient's skin integrity on admission to support the presence of a stage I pressure ulcer. However, the physician's documentation is unclear as to whether this condition was present on admission. How should the clinical documentation specialist proceed?

    a. Note the condition as present on admission

    b. Query the physician to determine if the condition was present on admission

    c. Note the condition as unknown on admission

    d. Note the condition as not present on admission

16. Mary Smith, RHIA, has been charged with the responsibility of designing a data collection form to be used on admission of a patient to the acute care hospital in which she works. The first resource that she should use is _____.

    a. UHDDS

    b. UACDS

    c. MDS

    d. ORYX

17. Both HEDIS and the Joint Commission's ORYX programs are designed to collect data to be used for _____.

    a. Performance improvement programs

    b. Billing and claims data processing

    c. Developing hospital discharge abstracting systems

    d. Developing individual care plans for residents

18. While the focus of inpatient data collection in the UHDDS is on principal diagnosis, the focus of outpatient data collection in the UACDS is on _____.

    a. Reason for admission

    b. Reason for encounter

    c. Discharge diagnosis

    d. Activities of daily living

19. In long-term care, the resident's care plan is based on data collected in the _____.

    a. UHDDS

    b. OASIS

    c. MDS Version 3.0

    d. HEDIS

20. A notation for a diabetic patient in a physician progress note reads: "Occasionally gets hungry. No insulin reactions. Says she is following her diabetic diet." In which part of a POMR progress note would this notation be written?

    a. Subjective

    b. Objective

    c. Assessment

    d. Plan

21. A notation for a diabetic patient in a physician progress note reads: "FBS 110 mg%, urine sugar, no acetone." In which part of a POMR progress note would this notation be written?

    a. Subjective

    b. Objective

    c. Assessment

    d. Plan

22. A notation for a hypertensive patient in a physician ambulatory care progress note reads: "Continue with Diuril, 500 mgs once daily. Return visit in 2 weeks." In which part of a POMR progress note would this notation be written?

    a. Subjective

    b. Objective

    c. Assessment

    d. Plan

23. A notation for a hypertensive patient in a physician ambulatory care progress note reads: "Blood pressure adequately controlled." In which part of a POMR progress note would this notation be written?

    a. Subjective

    b. Objective

    c. Assessment

    d. Plan

24. Which of the following provides the most comprehensive controlled vocabulary for coding the content of a patient record?

    a. CPT

    b. HCPCS

    c. ICD-9-CM

    d. SNOMED CT

25. Which of the following provides a set of codes used for collecting data about substance abuse and mental health disorders?

    a. CPT

    b. DSM-IV-TR

    c. HCPCS

    d. SNOMED CT

26. Dr. Jones entered a progress note in a patient's health record 24 hours after he visited the patient. Which quality element is missing from the progress note?

    a. Data completeness

    b. Data relevancy

    c. Data currency

    d. Data precision

27. The admitting data of Mrs. Smith's health record indicated that her birth date was March 21, 1948. On the discharge summary, Mrs. Smith's birth date was recorded as July 21, 1948. Which quality element is missing from Mrs. Smith's health record?

    a. Data completeness

    b. Data consistency

    c. Data accessibility

    d. Data comprehensiveness

28. The diagnosis of a patient was recorded as an abscess in the procedure report, but was listed as carcinoma on the discharge summary. This is an example of a problem with:

    a. Data granularity

    b. Data consistency

    c. Data precision

    d. Data relevance

29. Which of the following is an example of clinical data?

    a. Admitting diagnosis

    b. Date and time of admission

    c. Insurance information

    d. Health record number

30. Documentation of aides who assist a patient with activities of daily living, bathing, laundry, and cleaning would be found in which type of specialty record?

    a. Home health

    b. Behavioral health

    c. End stage renal disease

    d. Rehabilitative care

31. Which of the following materials is **not** documented in an emergency care record?

    a. Patient's instructions at discharge

    b. Time and means of the patient's arrival

    c. Patient's complete medical history

    d. Emergency care administered before arrival at the facility

32. Which of the following provides macroscopic and microscopic information about tissue removed during an operative procedure?

    a. Anesthesia report

    b. Laboratory report

    c. Operative report

    d. Pathology report

33. Sleeping patterns, head and chest measurements, feeding and elimination status, weight, and Apgar scores are recorded in which of the following records?

    a. Emergency

    b. Newborn

    c. Obstetric

    d. Surgical

34. In a problem-oriented medical record, problems are organized _____.

    a. In alphabetical order

    b. In numeric order

    c. In alphabetical order by body system

    d. By date of onset

35. What is the defining characteristic of an integrated health record format?

    a. Each section of the record is maintained by the patient care department that provided the care.

    b. Integrated health records are intended to be used in ambulatory settings.

    c. Integrated health records include both paper forms and computer printouts.

    d. Integrated health record components are arranged in strict chronological order.

36. Which of the following represents documentation of the patient's current and past health status?

    a. Physical exam

    b. Medical history

    c. Physician orders

    d. Patient consent

37. Which of the following contains the physician's findings based on an examination of the patient?

    a. Physical exam

    b. Discharge summary

    c. Medical history

    d. Patient instructions

38. What is the function of a consultation report?

    a. Provides a chronological summary of the patient's medical history and illness

    b. Documents opinions about the patient's condition from the perspective of a physician not previously involved in the patient's care

    c. Concisely summarizes the patient's treatment and stay in the hospital

    d. Documents the physician's instructions to other parties involved in providing care to a patient

39. What is the function of physician's orders?

    a. Provide a chronological summary of the patient's illness and treatment

    b. Document the patient's current and past health status

    c. Document the physician's instructions to other parties involved in providing care to a patient

    d. Document the provider's instructions for follow-up care given to the patient or patient's caregiver

40. Which type of patient care record includes documentation of a family bereavement period?

    a. Hospice record

    b. Home health record

    c. Long-term care record

    d. Ambulatory care record

Domain 2: Health Information Requirements and Standards

41. Which of the following best describes data completeness?

    a. Data are correct

    b. Data are easy to obtain

    c. Data include all required elements

    d. Data are reliable

42. The attending physician is responsible for which of the following types of acute care documentation?

    a. Consultation report

    b. Discharge summary

    c. Laboratory report

    d. Pathology report

43. A nurse is responsible for which of the following types of acute care documentation?

    a. Operative report

    b. Medication record

    c. Radiology report

    d. Therapy assessment

44. Reviewing the health record for missing signatures, missing medical reports, and ensuring that all documents belong in the health record is an example of _____ review.

    a. Quantitative

    b. Qualitative

    c. Statistical

    d. Outcomes

45. Which of the following is a secondary purpose of the health record?

    a. Support for provider reimbursement

    b. Support for patient self-management activities

    c. Support for research

    d. Support for patient care delivery

46. Use of the health record by a clinician to facilitate quality patient care is considered _____.

    a. A primary purpose of the health record

    b. Patient care support

    c. A secondary purpose of the health record

    d. Policy making and support

47. Use of the health record to monitor bioterrorism activity is considered a _____.

    a. Primary purpose of the health record

    b. Secondary purpose of the health record

    c. Patient use of the health record

    d. Healthcare licensing agency function

48. In designing an electronic health record, one of the best resources to use in helping to define the content of the record as well as to standardize data definitions is the E1384 standard promulgated by the:

    a. Centers for Medicare and Medicaid Services (CMS)

    b. American Society for Testing and Measurement (ASTM)

    c. Joint Commission

    d. National Centers for Health Statistics (NCHS)

49. The _____ mandated the development of standards for electronic medical records.

    a. Medicare and Medicaid legislation of 1965

    b. Prospective Payment Act of 1983

    c. Health Insurance Portability and Accountability Act (HIPAA) of 1996

    d. Balanced Budget Act of 1997

50. Messaging standards for electronic data interchange in healthcare have been developed by _____.

    a. HL7

    b. IEE

    c. The Joint Commission

    d. CMS

51. A statement or guideline that directs decision making or behavior is called a _____.

    a. Directive

    b. Procedure

    c. Policy

    d. Process

52. Which of the following is the planned replacement for ICD-9-CM Volumes 1 and 2?

    a. Current Procedural Terminology

    b. International Classification of Diseases, Ninth Revision, Clinical Modification

    c. International Classification of Diseases, Tenth Revision

    d. International Classification of Diseases, Tenth Revision, Clinical Modification

53. Which organization originally published ICD-9-CM?

    a. American Medical Association

    b. Centers for Disease Control

    c. United States federal government

    d. World Health Organization

54. Which of the following provides a system for coding the clinical procedures and services provided by physicians and other clinical professionals?

    a. Current Procedural Terminology

    b. Diagnostic and Statistical Manual of Mental Disorders, Fourth Revision

    c. Healthcare Common Procedure Coding System

    d. International Classification of Diseases, Ninth Revision, Clinical Modification

55. Which of the following is used to report the healthcare supplies, products, and services provided to patients by healthcare professionals?

    a. CPT

    b. HCPCS Level II

    c. ICD-9-CM

    d. SNOMED CT

56. A coding audit shows that an inpatient coder is using multiple codes that describe the individual components of a procedure rather than using a single code that describes all the steps of the procedure performed. Which of the following should be done in this case?

    a. Require all coders to implement this practice

    b. Report the practice to the OIG

    c. Counsel the coder and stop the practice immediately

    d. Put the coder on unpaid leave of absence

57. A health information technician is hired as the chief compliance officer for a large group practice. In evaluating the current program the HIT learns that there are written standards of conduct and policies and procedures that address specific areas of potential fraud as well as audits in place to monitor compliance. Which of the following should the compliance officer also ensure are in place?

    a. Compliance program education and training programs for all employees in the organization

    b. Establishment of a hotline to receive complaints and adoption of procedures to protect whistleblowers from retaliation

    c. Adopt procedures to adequately identify individuals who make complaints so that appropriate follow-up can be conducted

    d. Establish a corporate compliance committee who report directly to the CFO.

58. In developing a coding compliance program, which of the following would not be ordinarily included as participants in coding compliance education?

    a. Current coding personnel

    b. Medical staff

    c. Newly hired coding personnel

    d. Nursing staff

59. Which of the following issues compliance program guidance?

    a. AHIMA

    b. CMS

    c. Federal Register

    d. HHS Office of Inspector General

60. Which of the following is a written description of an organization's formal position?

    a. Hierarchy chart

    b. Organizational chart

    c. Policy

    d. Procedure

61. Community Hospital is launching a clinical documentation improvement initiative because currently clinical documentation does not always adequately reflect the severity of illness of the patient and does not support optimal HIM coding quality and accuracy. Given this situation, which of the following would be the **best** action to provide improved documentation for patient care and coding?

    a. Hire clinical documentation specialists to review records prior to coding.

    b. Ask coders to query physicians more often.

    c. Provide physicians the opportunity to add addenda to their reports to clarify documentation issues.

    d. Conduct qualitative analyses of inpatient records while the patient is hospitalized to identify opportunities to improve the documentation in the record.

62. The HIM department is planning to scan nonelectronic medical record documentation. The project includes the scanning of health record documentation such as history and physicals, physician orders, operative reports, and nursing notes. Which of the following methods of scanning would be best to help HIM professionals monitor the completeness of health records during a patient's hospitalization?

    a. Ad hoc

    b. Concurrent

    c. Retrospective

    d. Post-discharge

63. The inpatient data set that has been incorporated into federal law and is required for Medicare reporting is the _____.

    a. Ambulatory Care Data Set

    b. Uniform Hospital Discharge Data Set

    c. Minimum Data Set for Long-term Care

    d. Health Plan Employer Data and Information Set

64. What is it called when accrediting bodies such as the Joint Commission or American Osteopathic Association (AOA) Healthcare Facilities Accreditation Program can survey facilities for compliance with the Medicare Conditions of Participation for Hospitals instead of the government?

    a. Deemed status

    b. Judicial decision

    c. Subpoena

    d. Credentialing

65. Accreditation standards and the Medicare Conditions of Participation require that the patient's _____ be documented by the attending physician in the patient's health record no more than 30 days after discharge.

    a. Principal diagnosis

    b. Principal procedure

    c. Comorbidities

    d. Complications

66. What is the term used in reference to the systematic review of sample health records to determine whether health record documentation standards are being met?

    a. Qualitative analysis

    b. Legal record review

    c. Quantitative analysis

    d. Ongoing record review

67. The _____ notifies physicians that Medicare payment to the facility is partly based on the patient's principal and secondary diagnoses, as well as the major procedures performed, and that falsification of records can lead to fines, imprisonment, or civil penalty under federal laws.

    a. Medicare reimbursement rule

    b. Physician acknowledgment statement

    c. Provider agreement

    d. Diagnosis and procedure validation statement

68. Adoption of the Minimum Standards marked the beginning of this modern _____ process for healthcare organizations.

    a. Accreditation

    b. Licensing

    c. Reform

    d. Educational

Domain 3: Clinical Classification Systems

69. Identify the diagnosis code(s) for carcinoma in situ of vocal cord.

    a. 231.0

    b. 161.0

    c. 239.1

    d. 212.1

70. Identify the diagnosis code(s) for benign melanoma of skin of shoulder.

    a. 172.8, 172.6

    b. 172.6

    c. 172.9

    d. 172.8

71. Which of the following organizations is responsible for updating the procedure classification of ICD-9-CM?

    a. Centers for Disease Control (CDC)

    b. Centers for Medicare and Medicaid Services (CMS)

    c. National Center for Health Statistics (NCHS)

    d. World Health Organization (WHO)

72. At which level of the classification system are the most specific ICD-9-CM codes found?

    a. Category level

    b. Section level

    c. Subcategory level

    d. Subclassification level

73. What are five-digit ICD-9-CM diagnosis codes referred to as?

    a. Category codes

    b. Section codes

    c. Subcategory codes

    d. Subclassification codes

74. What are four-digit ICD-9-CM diagnosis codes referred to as?

    a. Category codes

    b. Section codes

    c. Subcategory codes

    d. Subclassification codes

75. Which of the following ICD-9-CM codes are always alphanumeric?

    a. Category codes

    b. Procedure codes

    c. Subcategory codes

    d. V codes

76. Which of the following ICD-9-CM codes classify environmental events and circumstances as the cause of an injury, poisoning, or other adverse effect?

    a. Category codes

    b. E codes

    c. Subcategory codes

    d. V codes

77. Which volume of ICD-9-CM contains the tabular and alphabetic lists of procedures?

    a. Volume 1

    b. Volume 2

    c. Volume 3

    d. Volume 4

78. Identify the correct diagnosis code for lipoma of the face.

    a. 214.1

    b. 213.0

    c. 214.0

    d. 214.9

79. Identify the correct diagnosis code(s) for adenoma of adrenal cortex with Conn's syndrome.

    a. 227.0, 255.12

    b. 227.0

    c. 255.12

    d. 225.12, 227.8

80. Which of the following is a standard terminology used to code medical procedures and services?

    a. CPT

    b. HCPCS

    c. ICD-9-CM

    d. SNOMED CT

81. Identify the appropriate ICD-9-CM diagnosis code for cerebral contusion with brief loss of consciousness.

    a. 924.9

    b. 851.42

    c. 851.82

    d. 851.81

82. If a patient has an excision of a malignant lesion of the skin, the CPT code is determined by the body area from which the excision occurs and which of the following?

    a. Length of the lesion as described in the pathology report

    b. Dimension of the specimen submitted as described in the pathology report

    c. Width times the length of the lesion as described in the operative report

    d. Diameter of the lesion as well as the most narrow margins required to adequately excise the lesion described in the operative report

83. According to CPT, a repair of a laceration that includes retention sutures would be considered what type of closure?

    a. Complex

    b. Intermediate

    c. Not specified

    d. Simple

84. The patient was admitted with nausea, vomiting, and abdominal pain. The physician documents the following on the discharge summary: acute cholecystitis, nausea, vomiting, and abdominal pain. Which of the following would be the correct coding and sequencing for this case?

    a. Acute cholecystitis, nausea, vomiting, abdominal pain

    b. Abdominal pain, vomiting, nausea, acute cholecystitis

    c. Nausea, vomiting, abdominal pain

    d. Acute cholecystitis

85. A patient is admitted with spotting. She had been treated two weeks previously for a miscarriage with sepsis. The sepsis had resolved and she is afebrile at this time. She is treated with an aspiration dilation and curettage. Products of conception are found. Which of the following should be the principal diagnosis?

    a. Miscarriage

    b. Complications of spontaneous abortion with sepsis

    c. Sepsis

    d. Spontaneous abortion with sepsis

86. An 80-year-old female is admitted with fever, lethargy, hypotension, tachycardia, oliguria, and elevated WBC. The patient has more than 100,000 organisms of *Escherichia coli* per cc of urine. The attending physician documents "urosepsis". How should the coder proceed to code this case?

    a. Code sepsis as the principal diagnosis with urinary tract infection due to *E. coli* as secondary diagnosis.

    b. Code urinary tract infection with sepsis as the principal diagnosis.

    c. Query the physician to ask if the patient has septicemia because of the symptomatology.

    d. Query the physician to ask if the patient had septic shock so that this may be used as the principal diagnosis.

87. A 65-year-old patient, with a history of lung cancer, is admitted to a healthcare facility with ataxia and syncope and a fractured arm as a result of falling. The patient undergoes a closed reduction of the fracture in the emergency department and undergoes a complete workup for metastatic carcinoma of the brain. The patient is found to have metastatic carcinoma of the lung to the brain and undergoes radiation therapy to the brain. Which of the following would be the principal diagnosis in this case?

    a. Ataxia

    b. Fractured arm

    c. Metastatic carcinoma of the brain

    d. Carcinoma of the lung

88. A patient was admitted for abdominal pain with diarrhea and was diagnosed with infectious gastroenteritis. The patient also has angina and chronic obstructive pulmonary disease. Which of the following would be the correct coding and sequencing for this case?

    a. Abdominal pain; infectious gastroenteritis; chronic obstructive pulmonary disease; angina

    b. Infectious gastroenteritis; chronic obstructive pulmonary disease; angina

    c. Gastroenteritis; abdominal pain; angina

    d. Gastroenteritis; abdominal pain; diarrhea; chronic obstructive pulmonary disease; angina

89. A patient is admitted with a history of prostate cancer and with mental confusion. The patient completed radiation therapy for prostatic carcinoma three years ago and is status post a radical resection of the prostate. A CT scan of the brain during the current admission reveals metastatic. Which of the following is the correct coding and sequencing for the current hospital stay?

    a. Metastatic carcinoma of the brain; carcinoma of the prostate; mental confusion

    b. Mental confusion; history of carcinoma of the prostate; admission for chemotherapy

    c. Metastatic carcinoma of the brain; history of carcinoma of the prostate

    d. Carcinoma of the prostate; metastatic carcinoma to the brain

90. A patient is admitted with abdominal pain. The physician states that the discharge diagnosis is pancreatitis versus noncalculus cholecystitis. Both diagnoses are equally treated. The correct coding and sequencing for this case would be:

    a. Sequence either the pancreatitis or noncalculus cholecystitis as principal diagnosis

    b. Pancreatitis; noncalculus cholecystitis; abdominal pain

    c. Noncalculus cholecystitis; pancreatitis; abdominal pain

    d. Abdominal pain; pancreatitis; noncalculus cholecystitis

91. According to the UHDDS, which of the following is the definition of "other diagnoses"?

    a. Is recorded in the patient record

    b. Is documented by the attending physician

    c. Receives clinical evaluation or therapeutic treatment or diagnostic procedures or extends the length of stay or increases nursing care and/or monitoring

    d. Is documented by at least two physicians and/or the nursing staff

92. A 7-year-old patient was admitted to the emergency department for treatment of shortness of breath. The patient is given epinephrine and nebulizer treatments. The shortness of breath and wheezing are unabated following treatment. What diagnosis should be suspected?

   a. Acute bronchitis

   b. Acute bronchitis with chronic obstructive pulmonary disease

   c. Asthma with status asthmaticus

   d. Chronic obstructive asthma

93. A patient was diagnosed with L4-5 lumbar neuropathy and discogenic pain. The patient underwent an intradiscal electrothermal annuloplasy (IDET) in the radiology suite. What ICD-9-CM code should be used?

   a. 80.50: Excision or destruction of intervertebral disc, unspecified

   b. 04.2: Destruction of cranial and peripheral nerves

   c. 80.59: Other destruction of intervertebral disc

   d. 05.23: Lumbar sympathectomy

94. A patient is seen in the emergency department for chest pain. After evaluation of the patient it is suspected that the patient may have gastroesophageal reflux disease (GERD). The final diagnosis was "Rule out chest pain versus GERD." The correct ICD-9-CM code is:

   a. V71.7, Admission for suspected cardiovascular condition

   b. 789.01, Esophageal pain

   c. 530.81, Gastrointestinal reflux

   d. 786.50, Chest pain NOS

95. A skin lesion is removed from a patient's cheek in the dermatologist's office. The dermatologist documents "skin lesion" in the health record. Prior to billing the pathology report returns with a diagnosis of basal cell carcinoma. Which of the following actions should the coding professional do for claim submission?

   a. Code skin lesion

   b. Code benign skin lesion

   c. Code basal cell carcinoma

   d. Query the dermatologist

96. An epidural was given during labor. Subsequently, it was determined that the patient would require a C-section for cephalopelvic disproportion because of obstructed labor. Assign the correct ICD-9-CM diagnostic and CPT anesthesia codes. (Modifiers are not used in this example.)

    a. 660.11, 653.41, 64475

    b. 660.11, 653.01, 01961

    c. 660.11, 653.41, 01967, 01968

    d. 660.11, 653.91, 01996

97. Dr. Smith sees his patient, Bob Jones, in the nursing home where he has resided for 11 months. Bob is stable and happy, and Dr. Smith performs an annual physical examination and completes the minimum data set instrument. He performs and documents a detailed interval history, comprehensive examination, and performs medical decision making of low complexity. Assign the appropriate CPT code.

    a. 99304

    b. 99308

    c. 99318

    d. 99306

98. A 61-year-old male patient is being assessed for possible colon cancer and treated in the special procedure unit of the hospital. He undergoes a colonoscopy into the ascending colon with biopsy of a suspicious area in the transverse colon using the cold biopsy forceps. In addition, a colonic ultrasound of the area is performed, with transmural biopsy of an area of the mesentery adjacent to the transverse colon. Assign the appropriate CPT codes.

    a. 45384, 45342

    b. 45380, 45391

    c. 45384, 45392

    d. 45380, 45392

99. Which of the following statements does not apply to ICD-9-CM?

    a. It can be used as the basis for epidemiological research.

    b. It can be used in the evaluation of medical care planning for healthcare delivery systems.

    c. It can be used to facilitate data storage and retrieval.

    d. It can be used to collect data about nursing care.

100. Which of the following is **not** one of the purposes of ICD-9-CM?

    a. Classification of morbidity for statistical purposes

    b. Classification of mortality for statistical purposes

    c. Reporting of diagnoses by physicians

    d. Identification of the supplies, products, and services provided to patients

101. Which volume of ICD-9-CM contains the numerical listing of codes that represent diseases and injuries?

    a. Volume 1

    b. Volume 2

    c. Volume 3

    d. Volume 4

102. When coding benign neoplasm of the skin, the section noted here directs the coder to:

216	Benign Neoplasm of Skin
	Includes:
	Blue Nevus
	Dermatofibroma
	Hydrocystoma
	Pigmented Nevus
	Syringoadenoma
	Syringoma
	Excludes:
	Skin of genital organs (221.0–222.9)
216.0	Skin of lip
	Excludes:
	Vermilion border of lip (210.0)
216.1	Eyelid, including canthus
	Excludes:
	Cartilage of eyelid (215.0)

    a. Use category 216 for syringoma.

    b. Use category 216 for malignant melanoma.

    c. Use category 216 for malignant neoplasm of the bone.

    d. Use category 216 for malignant neoplasm of the skin.

103. A 65-year-old patient is admitted with pain and loosening of a previous total hip arthroplasty. The acetabular component has loosened and become painful. The patient was admitted for revision of the hip replacement. The acetabular component uses a metal-on-metal bearing surface. Which of the following codes would be the appropriate coding for the admission?

996.41	Mechanical loosening of prosthetic joint
996.96	Infection and inflammatory reaction to joint prosthesis
V43.64	Organ or tissue replaced by other means
00.71	Revision hip replacement, acetabular component
00.74	Revision hip replacement bearing surface, metal on polyethylene
00.75	Revision hip replacement bearing surface, metal on metal
00.76	Revision hip replacement bearing surface, ceramic on ceramic

a. 996.41, V43.64, 00.71, 00.75

b. 996.96, 00.75

c. 996.41, V43.64, 00.71

d. 996.96, V43.64, 00.71, 00.75

104. A patient was discharged with the following diagnoses: "Cerebral occlusion, hemiparesis, asphasia, and hypertension." Which of the following code assignments would be appropriate for this case?

342.90	Hemiparesis affecting unspecified side
342.91	Hemiparesis affecting dominant side
342.92	Hemiparesis affecting nondominant side
434.90	Cerebral artery occlusion unspecified, without mention of cerebral infarction
434.91	Cerebral artery occlusion unspecified with cerebral infarction
401	Hypertension
401.0	Malignant hypertension
401.1	Benign hypertension
401.9	Unspecified hypertension
428.0	Congestive heart failure
784.3	Aphasia

a. 434.91, 342.92, 784.3, 401

b. 434.90, 342.90, 784.3, 401.9

c. 434.90, 342.91, 784.3, 401.9

d. 434.90, 342.90, 784.3, 401.0

105. CPT codes describing endovascular repair of the descending thoracic aorta include all of the following procedures except one. Which procedure is not included in the repair code?

   a. Intravascular ultrasound

   b. Angiography of the thoracic aorta

   c. Fluoroscopic guidance in delivery of the endovascular components

   d. Preprocedure diagnostic imaging

106. A patient is admitted to the hospital with shortness of breath and congestive heart failure. The patient subsequently develops respiratory failure. The patient undergoes intubation with ventilator management. Which of the following would be the correct sequencing and coding of this case?

   a. Congestive heart failure, respiratory failure, ventilator management, intubation

   b. Respiratory failure, intubation, ventilator management

   c. Respiratory failure, congestive heart failure, intubation, ventilator management

   d. Shortness of breath, congestive heart failure, respiratory failure, ventilator management

107. A physician correctly prescribes Coumadin. The patient takes the Coumadin as prescribed, but develops hematuria as a result of taking the medication. Which of the following is the correct way to code this case?

   a. Poisoning due to Coumadin

   b. Unspecified adverse reaction to Coumadin

   c. Hematuria; poisoning due to Coumadin

   d. Hematuria; adverse reaction to Coumadin

108. CPT Category III codes can be used by what groups of providers?

   a. Hospital outpatient providers only

   b. Physicians only

   c. Hospitals, physicians, insurers, health services researchers

   d. Medicare-approved providers only

109. A patient is admitted for chest pain with cardiac dysrhythmia to Hospital A. The patient is found to have an acute inferior myocardial infarction with atrial fibrillation. After the atrial fibrillation was controlled and the patient was stabilized, the patient was transferred to Hospital B for a CABG X3. Using the codes listed here, what are the appropriate ICD-9-CM codes and sequencing for both hospitalizations?

410.00	Myocardial infarction of anterolateral wall, episode unspecified
410.01	Myocardial infarction of anterolateral wall, initial episode
410.40	Myocardial infarction of inferior wall, episode unspecified
410.41	Myocardial infarction of inferior wall, initial episode
410.42	Myocardial infarction of inferior wall, subsequent episode
427	Cardiac dysrhythmias
427.3	Atrial fibrillation and flutter
427.31	Atrial fibrillation
786.50	Chest pain, unspecified
36.13	Aortocoronary bypass of three coronary arteries

    a. Hospital A: 427, 786.50, 427.31, 410.91; Hospital B: 410.92, 36.13

    b. Hospital A: 410.41, 427, 427.31; Hospital B: 410.42, 36.13

    c. Hospital A: 410.41, 427.31; Hospital B: 410.41, 36.13

    d. Hospital A: 410.41, 427.31, 786.50; Hospital B: 410.42, 36.13

110. A patient is admitted to the hospital with abdominal pain. The principal diagnosis is cholecystitis. The patient also has a history of hypertension and diabetes. In the DRG prospective payment system, which of the following would determine the MDC assignment for this patient?

    a. Abdominal pain

    b. Cholecystitis

    c. Hypertension

    d. Diabetes

111. A patient was admitted to the hospital with symptoms of a stroke and secondary diagnoses of COPD and hypertension. The patient was subsequently discharged from the hospital with a principal diagnosis of cerebral vascular accident and secondary diagnoses of catheter-associated urinary tract infection, COPD, and hypertension. Which of the following diagnoses should **not** be tagged as POA?

    a. Catheter-associated urinary tract infection

    b. Cerebral vascular accident

    c. COPD

    d. Hypertension

112. Which of the following is a condition that arises during hospitalization?

    a. Case mix

    b. Complication

    c. Comorbidity

    d. Principal diagnosis

113. A 65-year-old woman was admitted to the hospital. She was diagnosed with septicemia secondary to staphylococcus aureus and abdominal pain secondary to diverticulitis of the colon. What is the correct code assignment?

    a. 038.8, 562.11, 789.00

    b. 038.11, 562.11

    c. 038.8, 562.11, 041.11

    d. 038.9, 562.11

114. Patient had carcinoma of the anterior bladder wall fulgurated three years ago. The patient returns yearly for a cystoscopy to recheck for bladder tumor. Patient is currently admitted for a routine check. A small recurring malignancy is found and fulgurated during the cystoscopy procedure. Which is the correct code assignment?

    a. 188.3; V10.51; 57.49; 57.32

    b. 198.1; 57.49

    c. 188.3; 57.49

    d. 198.1; 188.3; 57.49

115. A patient with a diagnosis of ventral hernia is admitted to undergo a laparotomy with ventral hernia repair. The patient undergoes a laparotomy and develops bradycardia. The operative site is closed without the repair of the hernia, which is the correct code assignment?

    a. 553.20; 427.89; V64.3; 54.11

    b. 553.20; 997.1; 427.89; 54.19

    c. 553.20; 54.11

    d. 553.20; 54.11; V64.3

116. These codes are used to assign a diagnosis to a patient who is seeking health services, but is not necessarily sick.

    a. E codes

    b. V codes

    c. M codes

    d. C codes

117. Patient was admitted through the emergency department following a fall from a ladder while painting an interior room in his house. He had contusions of the scalp and face and an open fracture of the acetabulum. The fracture site was débrided and the fracture was reduced by open procedure with an external fixation device applied, which is the correct code assignment?

    a. 808.1; E881.0, E849.0; 79.25; 78.15

    b. 808.1; 920; E881.0; E849.0; E000.8, E013.9, 79.25; 78.15; 79.65

    c. 808.0; E881.0; E000.8, E013.9, 79.35; 79.65

    d. 808.1; E881.0; E849.0; E013.9, 79.25; 78.15; 79.65

118. Assign the correct CPT code for the following procedure: Revision of the pacemaker skin pocket:

    a. 33223

    b. 33210

    c. 33212

    d. 33222

119. Assign the correct CPT code for the following: A 58-year-old male was seen in the outpatient surgical center for an insertion of self-contained inflatable penile prosthesis for impotence.

    a. 54401

    b. 54405

    c. 54440

    d. 54400

120. Patient returns during a 90-day postoperative period from a ventral hernia repair; now complaining of eye pain. What modifier would a physician setting use with the Evaluation and Management code?

    a. −79: Unrelated procedure or service by the same physician during the postoperative period

    b. −25: Significant, separately identifiable evaluation and management service by the same physician on the same day of the procedure or other service

    c. −21: Prolonged evaluation and management services

    d. −24: Unrelated evaluation and management service by the same physician during a postoperative period

121. A patient is admitted to an acute care hospital for acute intoxication and alcohol withdrawal syndrome due to chronic alcoholism.

    a. 291.8; 303.00

    b. 303.00

    c. 305.00

    d. 291.81; 303.00

122. A 45-year-old woman is admitted for blood loss anemia due to dysfunctional uterine bleeding.

    a. 280.0; 626.8

    b. 285.1; 626.8

    c. 626.8; 280.0

    d. 280.0; 218.9

123. Patient admitted with senile cataract, diabetes mellitus, and extracapsular cataract extraction with simultaneous insertion of intraocular lens.

    a. 366.10; 250.50; 13.59; 13.71

    b. 250.00; 366.10

    c. 250.00; 366.12

    d. 366.10; 250.00; 13.59; 13.71

124. A patient is admitted with acute exacerbation of COPD, chronic renal failure, and hypertension.

    a. 492.8; 496; 403.10, 585.9

    b. 492.8; 585.9; 401.9

    c. 496; 585.9; 401.9

    d. 491.21; 403.91, 585.9

125. Patient arrived via ambulance to the emergency department following a motor vehicle accident. Patient sustained a fracture of the ankle; 3.0 cm superficial laceration of the left arm; 5.0 laceration of the scalp with exposure of the fascia; and a concussion. Patient received the following procedures: X-ray of the ankle which showed a bimalleolar ankle fracture which required closed manipulative reduction and simple suturing of the laceration. Provide CPT codes for the procedures done in the emergency department for the facility bill.

    a. 27810, 12032

    b. 27818, 12032

    c. 27810, 12032, 12002

    d. 27810, 12032

126. The patient was admitted to the outpatient department and had a bronchoscopy with bronchial brushings performed:

    a. 31622, 31640

    b. 31622, 31623

    c. 31623

    d. 31625

127. Identify the two-digit modifier that may be reported to indicate a physician performed the postoperative management of a patient, but another physician performed the surgical procedure.

    a. 22

    b. 54

    c. 32

    d. 55

128. What is the correct CPT code assignment for destruction of internal hemorrhoids with use of infrared coagulation?

    a. 46255

    b. 46930

    c. 46260

    d. 46945

129. An encoder that takes a coder through a series of questions and choices is called a(n):

    a. Automated codebook

    b. Automated code assignment

    c. Logic-based encoder

    d. Decision support database

130. Patient admitted with major depression, recurrent, severe.

    a. 296.33

    b. 296.30

    c. 311

    d. 296.89

131. A 35-year-old male was admitted with esophageal reflux. An esophagoscopy and closed esophageal biopsy was performed. Identify the code for the ICD-9-CM diagnosis and procedure.

    a. 530.89; 49.29

    b. 530.1; 45.16

    c. 530.81; 42.24

    d. 530.81; 42.23

132. Patient with flank pain was admitted and found to have a calculus of the kidney. Ureteroscopy with placement of ureteral stents was performed.

    a. 592.0; 788.0; 59.8

    b. 788.0; 592.0; 56.0

    c. 594.9; 59.8

    d. 592.0; 59.8

133. A female patient is admitted for stress incontinence. A urethral suspension is performed.

    a. 625.6; 57.32

    b. 788.0; 59.5

    c. 625.6; 59.5

    d. 788.30

134. Reference codes 49491 through 49525 for inguinal hernia repair. Patient is 47 years old. What is the correct code for an initial inguinal herniorrhaphy for incarcerated hernia?

    a. 49496

    b. 49501

    c. 49507

    d. 49521

135. Patient had a laparoscopic incisional herniorrhaphy for a recurrent reducible hernia. The repair included insertion of mesh. What is the correct code assignment?

    a. 49565

    b. 49565, 49568

    c. 49656

    d. 49560, 49568

136. What is the correct CPT code assignment for hysteroscopy with lysis of intrauterine adhesions?

    a. 58555, 58559

    b. 58559

    c. 58559, 58740

    d. 58555, 58559, 58740

137. The physician performs an exploratory laparotomy with bilateral salpingo-oophorectomy. What is the correct CPT code assignment for this procedure?

    a. 49000, 58940, 58700

    b. 58940, 58720–50

    c. 49000, 58720

    d. 58720

138. Identify the CPT code for a 42-year-old diagnosed with ESRD who requires home dialysis for the month of April.

    a. 90965

    b. 90964

    c. 90966

    d. 90970

139. Identify the appropriate CPT code(s) for a routine EKG with 15 leads, with the physician providing only the interpretation and report.

    a. 93010

    b. 93005

    c. 93000

    d. 93000; 93010

140. The patient presented to the physical therapy department and received 30 minutes of water aerobics therapeutic exercise with the therapist for treatment of arthritis. What is the appropriate treatment code(s) and/or modifier for a Medicare patient on a physical therapy plan of care in an outpatient setting?

    a. 97113

    b. 97113–50

    c. 97113; 97113

    d. 97110

Domain 4: Reimbursement Methodologies

141. Given the following information, which of the following statements is correct?

MS-DRG	MDC	Type	MS-DRG Title	Weight	Discharges	Geometric Mean	Arithmetic Mean
191	04	MED	Chronic obstructive pulmonary disease w CC	0.9757	10	4.1	5.0
192	04	MED	Chronic obstructive pulmonary disease w/o CC/MCC	0.7254	20	3.3	4.0
193	04	MED	Simple pneumonia & pleurisy w MCC	1.4327	10	5.4	6.7
194	04	MED	Simple pneumonia & pleurisy w CC	1.0056	20	4.4	5.3
195	04	MED	Simple pneumonia & pleurisy w/o CC/MCC	0.7316	10	3.5	4.1

a. In each MS-DRG the geometric mean is lower than the arithmetic mean.

b. In each MS-DRG the arithmetic mean is lower than the geometric mean.

c. The higher the number of patients in each MS-DRG, the greater the geometric mean for that MS-DRG.

d. The geometric means are lower in MS-DRGs that are associated with a CC or MCC.

142. If another status T procedure were performed, how much would the facility receive for the second status T procedure?

Billing Number	Status Indicator	CPT/HCPCS	APC
998323	V	99285–25	0612
998324	T	25500	0044
998325	X	72050	0261
998326	S	72128	0283
998327	S	70450	0283

   a. 0 percent

   b. 50 percent

   c. 75 percent

   d. 100 percent

143. A health information technician is processing payments for hospital outpatient services to be reimbursed by Medicare for a patient who had two physician visits, underwent radiology examinations, clinical laboratory tests, and who received take-home surgical dressings. Which of the following could be reimbursed under the outpatient prospective payment system?

   a. Clinical laboratory tests

   b. Physician office visits

   c. Radiology examinations

   d. Take-home surgical dressings

144. Which of the following types of hospitals are excluded from the Medicare inpatient prospective payment system?

   a. Children's

   b. Rural

   c. State supported

   d. Tertiary

145. Diagnosis-related groups are organized into _____.

   a. Case-mix classifications

   b. Geographic practice cost indices

   c. Major diagnostic categories

   d. Resource-based relative values

146. In processing a Medicare payment for outpatient radiology exams, a hospital outpatient services department would receive payment under which of the following?

    a. DRGs

    b. HHRGS

    c. OASIS

    d. OPPS

147. Which of the following is **not** reimbursed according to the Medicare outpatient prospective payment system?

    a. CMHC partial hospitalization services

    b. Critical access hospitals

    c. Hospital outpatient departments

    d. Vaccines provided by CORFs

148. Fee schedules are updated by third-party payers _____.

    a. Annually

    b. Monthly

    c. Semiannually

    d. Weekly

149. Which of the following would a health record technician use to perform the billing function for a physician's office?

    a. CMS-1500

    b. UB-04

    c. UB-92

    d. CMS 1450

150. When a provider accepts assignment, this means the _____.

    a. Patient authorizes payment to be made directly to the provider

    b. The provider agrees to accept the allowed payment amount by the payer as payment in full for the items or service

    c. Balance filling is allowed on patient accounts, but at a limited rate

    d. Participating provider receives a fee-for-service reimbursement

151. A coding audit shows that an inpatient coder is using multiple codes that describe the individual components of a procedure rather than using a single code that describes all the steps of the procedure performed. Which of the following should be done in this case?

    a. Require all coders to implement this practice

    b. Report the practice to the OIG

    c. Counsel the coder and stop the practice immediately

    d. Put the coder on unpaid leave of absence

152. Prospective payment systems were developed by the federal government to:

    a. Increase healthcare access

    b. Manage Medicare and Medicaid costs

    c. Implement managed care programs

    d. Eliminate fee-for-service programs

153. Given NCCI edits, if the placement of a catheter is billed along with the performance of an infusion procedure for the same date of service for an outpatient beneficiary, Medicare will pay for:

    a. The placement of the catheter

    b. The placement of the catheter and the infusion procedure

    c. The infusion procedure

    d. Neither the placement of the catheter nor the infusion procedure

154. The goal of coding compliance programs is to prevent _____.

    a. Accusations of fraud and abuse

    b. Delays in claims processing

    c. Billing errors

    d. Inaccurate code assignments

155. Which of the following actions would be **best** to determine if present on admission (POA) indicators for the conditions selected by CMS are having a negative impact on the hospital's Medicare reimbursement?

    a. Identify all records for a period having these indicators for these conditions and determine if these conditions are the only secondary diagnosis present on the claim that will lead to higher payment.

    b. Identify all records for a period that have these indicators for these conditions.

    c. Identify all records for a period that have these indicators for these conditions and determine whether or not additional documentation can be submitted to Medicare to increase reimbursement.

    d. Take a random sample of records for a period of records having these indicators for these conditions and extrapolate the negative impact on Medicare reimbursement.

156. From the information provided, how many APCs would this patient have?

Billing Number	Status Indicator	CPT/HCPCS	APC
998323	V	99285–25	0612
998324	T	25500	0044
998325	X	72050	0261
998326	S	72128	0283
998327	S	70450	0283

a. 1

b. 4

c. 5

d. 3

157. If a patient's total outpatient bill is $500, and the patient's healthcare insurance plan pays 80 percent of the allowable charges, what is the amount for which the patient is responsible?

a. $10

b. $40

c. $100

d. $400

158. In a managed fee-for service arrangement, which of the following would be used as a cost-control process for inpatient surgical services?

a. Prospectively precertify the necessity of inpatient services

b. Determine what services can be bundled

c. Pay only 80 percent of the inpatient bill

d. Require the patient to pay 20 percent of the inpatient bill

159. The sum of a hospital's relative DRG rates for a year was 15,192 and the hospital had 10,471 discharges for the year. Given this information what would be the hospital's case-mix index for that year?

a. 0.689

b. 0.689 × 100

c. 1.45 × 100

d. 1.45

160. In processing a bill under the Medicare outpatient prospective payment system (OPPS), where a patient had three surgical procedures performed during the same operative session, which of the following would apply?

    a. Bundling of services

    b. Outlier adjustment

    c. Pass-through payment

    d. Discounting of procedures

Domain 5: Information and Communication Technologies

161. Which of the following is **not** an element of data quality?

    a. Accessibility

    b. Data back up

    c. Precision

    d. Relevancy

162. The protection measures and tools for safeguarding information and information systems is a definition of:

    a. Confidentiality

    b. Data security

    c. Informational privacy

    d. Informational access control

163. Computer software programs that assist in the assignment of codes used with diagnostic and procedural classifications are called _____.

    a. Natural language processing systems

    b. Monitoring/audit programs

    c. Encoders

    d. Concept, description, and relationship tables

164. A special Web page that offers secure access to data is called a(n):

    a. Access control

    b. Home page

    c. Intranet

    d. Portal

165. Which of the following technologies would allow a hospital to get as much medical record information online as quickly as possible?

   a. Clinical data repository

   b. Picture archiving system

   c. Electronic document management system

   d. Speech recognition system

166. Which of the following is necessary to ensure that each term used in an EHR has a common meaning to all users?

   a. Encoded vocabulary

   b. Controlled vocabulary

   c. Data exchange standards

   d. Proprietary standards

167. Which of the following tasks may **not** be performed in an electronic health record system?

   a. Document imaging

   b. Analysis

   c. Assembly

   d. Indexing

168. Electronic systems used by nurses and physicians to document assessments and findings are called:

   a. Computerized provider order entry

   b. Electronic document management systems

   c. Electronic medication administration record

   d. Electronic patient care charting

169. Data definition refers to _____.

   a. Meaning of data

   b. Completeness of data

   c. Consistency of data

   d. Detail of data

170. In the relational database here the patient table and the visit table are related by _____.

Patient Table			
Patient #	Patient Last Name	Patient First Name	Date of Birth
021234	Smith	Donna	03/21/1944
022366	Jones	William	04/09/1960
034457	Collins	Mary	08/21/1977

Visit Table			
Visit #	Date of Visit	Practitioner #	Patient #
0045678	11/12/2008	456	021234
0045679	11/12/2008	997	021234
0045680	11/12/2008	456	034457

a. Visit number

b. Date of visit

c. Patient number

d. Practitioner number

171. The ability to electronically send data from one electronic system to a different electronic system and still retain its meaning is called _____.

a. Data comparability

b. National data exchange

c. Interoperability

d. Data architecture

172. The key data element for linking data about an individual who is seen in a variety of care settings is the _____.

a. Facility medical record number

b. Facility identification number

c. Unique patient identifier

d. Patient birth date

Domain 6: Privacy, Confidentiality, Legal, and Ethical Issues

173. What is the legal term used to define the protection of health information in a patient–provider relationship?

    a. Access

    b. Confidentiality

    c. Privacy

    d. Security

174. The Uniform Health Care Decisions Act ranks the next-of-kin in the following order for medical decision-making purposes:

    a. Adult sibling; adult child; spouse; parent

    b. Parent; spouse; adult child; adult sibling

    c. Spouse; parent; adult sibling; adult child

    d. Spouse; adult child; parent; adult sibling

175. Which of the following is a direct command that requires an individual or a representative of an organization to appear in court or to present an object to the court?

    a. Judicial decision

    b. Subpoena

    c. Credential

    d. Regulation

176. Employees in the Hospital Business Office may have legitimate access to patient health information without patient authorization based on what HIPAA standard/principle?

    a. Minimum necessary

    b. Compound authorization

    c. Accounting of disclosures

    d. Preemption

177. Exceptions to the consent requirement include:

    a. Medical emergencies

    b. Provider discretion

    c. Implied consent

    d. Informed consent

178. Which of the following is required in order to prescribe medications?

    a. Active medical staff membership

    b. A drug enforcement agency number

    c. A position on a medical staff executive committee

    d. A credential from a nationally recognized association

179. Which of the following must be reported to the medical examiner?

    a. Burns

    b. Accidental deaths

    c. Causes of injury

    d. Morbidity

180. Dr. Williams is on the medical staff of Sutter Hospital and he has asked to see the health record of his wife who was recently hospitalized. Dr. Jones was the patient's physician. Of the options listed here, which is the **best** course of action?

    a. Refer Dr. Williams to Dr. Jones and release the record if Dr. Jones agrees.

    b. Inform Dr. Williams that he cannot access his wife's health information unless she authorizes access through a written release of information.

    c. Request that Dr. Williams ask the hospital administrator for approval to access his wife's record.

    d. Inform Dr. Williams that he may review his wife's health record in the presence of the privacy officer.

181. Under HIPAA rules, when an individual asks to see his or her own health information, a covered entity _____.

    a. Must always provide access

    b. Can deny access to psychotherapy notes

    c. Can demand that the individual pay to see his or her record

    d. Can always deny access

182. The legal health record is a(n) _____.

    a. Defined subset of all patient-specific data created or accumulated by a healthcare provider that may be released to third parties in response to a legally permissible request for patient information

    b. Entire set of information created or accumulated by a healthcare provider that may be released to third parties in response to a legally permissible request for patient information

    c. Set of patient-specific data created or accumulated by a healthcare provider that is defined to be legal by the local, state, or federal authorities

    d. Set of patient-specific data that is defined to be legal by state or federal statute and that is legally permissible to provide in response to requests for patient information

183. Privacy can be defined as the _____.

    a. Limitation of the use and disclosure of private information

    b. Right of an individual to be left alone

    c. Physical and electronic protection of information

    d. Protection of information from accidental or intentional disclosure

184. Which of the following statements represents an example of nonmaleficence?

    a. HITs must ensure that patient-identifiable information is not released to unauthorized parties.

    b. HITs must apply rules fairly and consistently to every case.

    c. HITs must ensure that patient-identifiable information is released to the parties who need it to provide services to their patients.

    d. HITs must ensure that patients themselves, and not other parties, are authorizing access to the patients' individual health information.

185. Attorneys for healthcare organizations use the health record to _____.

    a. Support claims for medical malpractice

    b. Protect the legal interests of the facility and its healthcare providers

    c. Plan and market services

    d. Locate missing persons

186. Which of the following federal laws passed in 1996 resulted in new privacy regulations for healthcare organizations?

    a. Health Information Access and Disclosure Act

    b. Health Insurance Portability and Accountability Act

    c. Patient Self-Determination Act

    d. Social Security Act

187. Written or spoken permission to proceed with care is classified as _____.

    a. An advanced directive

    b. Formal consent

    c. Expressed consent

    d. Implied consent

188. To be in compliance with HIPAA regulations, a hospital would make its membership in a RHIO known to its patients through which of the following?

    a. Press release

    b. Notice of Privacy Practices

    c. Consent form

    d. Web site notice

189. The number that has been proposed for use as a unique patient identification number but is controversial because of confidentiality and privacy concerns is the _____.

    a. Social security number

    b. Unique physician identification number

    c. Health record number

    d. National provider identifier

190. In which setting may treatment records travel with the patient between treatment centers?

    a. Ambulatory care

    b. Behavioral healthcare

    c. Correctional facility care

    d. Long-term care

191. Which of the following dictates how the medical staff operates?

    a. Medical staff classification

    b. Medical staff bylaws

    c. Medical staff credentialing

    d. Medical staff committees

192. Law enacted by a legislative body is a(n) _____.

    a. Administrative law

    b. Statute

    c. Regulation

    d. Rule

193. Which stage of the litigation process focuses on how strong a case the opposing party has?

   a. Deposition

   b. Discovery

   c. Trial

   d. Verdict

194. Which of the following is **not** true of notices of privacy practices?

   a. They must be made available at the site where the individual is treated.

   b. They must be posted in a prominent place.

   c. They must contain content that may not be changed.

   d. They must be prominently posted on the covered entity's Web site when the entity has one.

195. Which of the following spells out the powers of the three branches of the federal government?

   a. United States Constitution

   b. Statutes

   c. Administrative law

   d. Judicial decisions

196. Which document directs an individual to bring originals or copies of records to court?

   a. Summons

   b. Subpoena

   c. Subpoena *duces tecum*

   d. Deposition

197. To comply with HIPAA, under usual circumstances, a covered entity must act on a patient's request to review or copy his or her health information within _____ days.

   a. 10

   b. 20

   c. 30

   d. 60

198. The HIPAA Privacy Rule requires that covered entities must limit use, access, and disclosure of PHI to only the amount needed to accomplish the intended purpose. What concept is this an example of?

a. Minimum Necessary

b. Notice of Privacy Practices

c. Authorization

d. Consent

199. Which of the following statements is **false**?

a. A notice of privacy practices must be written in plain language.

b. A consent for use and disclosure of information must be obtained from every patient.

c. An authorization does not have to be obtained for uses and disclosures for treatment, payment, and operations.

d. A notice of privacy practices must give an example of a use or disclosure for healthcare operations.

200. Which of the following statements is **not** true about a business associate agreement?

a. It prohibits the business associate from using or disclosing PHI for any purpose other than that described in the contract with the covered entity.

b. It allows the business associate to maintain PHI indefinitely.

c. It prohibits the business associate from using or disclosing PHI in any way that would violate the HIPAA Privacy Rule.

d. It requires the business associate to make available all of its books and records relating to PHI use and disclosure to the Department of Health and Human Services or its agents.

Certified Coding Associate
Exam Preparation

Exam 1

Domain 1: Health Records and Data Content

1. An outpatient clinic is reviewing the functionality of a computer system it is considering purchasing. Which of the following datasets should the clinic consult to ensure all the federally required data elements for Medicare and Medicaid outpatient clinical encounters are collected by the system?

   a. DEEDS

   b. EMEDS

   c. UACDS

   d. UHDDS

2. Standardizing medical terminology to avoid differences in naming various medical conditions and procedures (such as the synonyms bunionectomy, McBride procedure, and repair of hallus valgus) is one purpose of _____.

   a. Transaction standards

   b. Content and structure standards

   c. Vocabulary standards

   d. Security standards

3. A family practitioner requests the opinion of a physician specialist in endocrinology who reviews the patient's health record and examines the patient. The physician specialist would record findings, impressions, and recommendations in which type of report?

   a. Consultation

   b. Medical history

   c. Physical examination

   d. Progress notes

4. Which of the following is **not** a function of the discharge summary?

   a. Providing information about the patient's insurance coverage

   b. Ensuring the continuity of future care

   c. Providing information to support the activities of the medical staff review committee

   d. Providing concise information that can be used to answer information requests

5. Ensuring the continuity of future care by providing information to the patient's attending physician, referring physician, and any consulting physicians is a function of the:

   a. Discharge summary

   b. Autopsy report

   c. Incident report

   d. Consent to treatment

6. A 65-year-old white male was admitted to the hospital on 1/15 complaining of abdominal pain. The Attending physician requested an upper GI series and laboratory evaluation of CBC and UA. The x-ray revealed possible cholelithiasis and the UA showed an increased white blood cell count. The patient was taken to surgery for an exploratory laparoscopy and a ruptured appendix was discovered. The chief complaint was:

   a. Ruptured appendix

   b. Exploratory laparoscopy

   c. Abdominal pain

   d. Cholelithiasis

7. All documentation entered in the medical record relating to the patient's diagnosis and treatment are considered this type of data:

   a. Clinical

   b. Identification

   c. Secondary

   d. Financial

8. What type of data is exemplified by the insured party's member identification number?

   a. Demographic data

   b. Clinical data

   c. Certification data

   d. Financial data

9. Which part of the problem-oriented medical record is used by many facilities that have not adopted the whole problem-oriented format?

   a. The problem list as an index

   b. The initial plan

   c. The SOAP form of progress notes

   d. The database

10. While the focus of inpatient data collection is on the principal diagnosis, the focus of outpatient data collection is on _____.

    a. Reason for admission

    b. Reason for encounter

    c. Discharge diagnosis

    d. Activities of daily living

11. Mildred Smith was admitted from an acute hospital to a nursing facility with the following information: "Patient is being admitted for Organic Brain Syndrome". Underneath the diagnosis was listed her medical information along with her rehabilitation potential. On which form is this information documented?

    a. Transfer or referral

    b. Release of information

    c. Patients rights acknowledgement

    d. Admitting physical evaluation

12. The coder notes that the physician has prescribed Synthroid for the patient. The coder might find which of the following on the patient's problem list?

    a. Acromegaly

    b. Hypothyroidism

    c. Dwarfism

    d. Cushing's disease

13. A male patient is seen by the physician and diagnosed with pneumonia. The doctor took cultures to try to determine which organism was causing the pneumonia. Which of the following organisms would alert the coder to code it as a gram-negative pneumonia?

    a. Staphylococcus

    b. Clostridium

    c. Klebsiella

    d. Streptococcus

14. What is the **best** source of documentation to determine the size of a removed malignant lesion?

    a. Pathology report

    b. Postacute care unit record

    c. Operative report

    d. Physical examination

15. The coder might find which of the following on a patient's problem list if the medication list contains the drug Protonix?

    a. High blood pressure

    b. Esophagitis

    c. Congestive heart failure

    d. AIDS

16. The patient is seen in the physician office with a chief complaint of shortness of breath. In the patient's progress notes, the physician documents the diagnosis of asthma and recommends the patient present to the emergency department of XYZ Hospital immediately. The physician further documents that the patient has severe wheezing and no obvious relief with bronchodilators. Which action will the coder take?

    a. Code asthma

    b. Code asthma with status asthmaticus

    c. Code asthma with acute exacerbation

    d. Query the physician for more detail about the asthma

17. The coder notes that the physician has ordered potassium replacement for the patient. The coder might expect to see a diagnosis of:

    a. Hypokalemia

    b. Hyponatremia

    c. Hyperkalemia

    d. Hypernatremia

18. The _____ may contain information about diseases among relatives in which heredity may play a role.

    a. Physical examination

    b. History

    c. Laboratory report

    d. Administrative data

19. The physician orders a chest x-ray for a patient who presents at the office with fever, productive cough, and shortness of breath. The physician indicates in the progress notes: "Rule out pneumonia." What diagnosis(es) should be coded for the visit when the results have not yet been received?

    a. Pneumonia

    b. Fever, cough, shortness of breath

    c. Cough, shortness of breath

    d. Pneumonia, cough, shortness of breath

20. Which term describes the linking of every procedure or service received by a patient to a diagnosis that justifies the need for performing the service?

    a. Medical necessity

    b. Managed care

    c. Medical decision making

    d. Level of services

Domain 2: Health Information Requirements and Standards

21. To comply with Joint Commission standards, the HIM director wants to ensure that history and physical examinations are documented in the patient's health record no later than 24 hours after admission. Which of the following would be the best way to ensure the completeness of health records?

    a. Retrospectively review each patient's medical record to make sure history and physicals are present

    b. Review each patient's medical record concurrently to make sure history and physicals are present and meet the accreditation standards

    c. Establish a process to review medical records immediately on discharge

    d. Do a review of records for all patients discharged in the previous 60 days

22. Medical record completion compliance is a problem at Community Hospital. The number of incomplete charts often exceed the standard set by the Joint Commission, risking a type I violation. Previous HIM committee chairpersons tried multiple methods to improve compliance, including suspension of privileges and deactivating the parking garage keycard of any physician in poor standing. To improve compliance, which of the following would be a next step to overcoming noncompliance?

    a. Discuss the problem with the hospital CEO

    b. Call the Joint Commission

    c. Contact other hospitals to see what methods they use to ensure compliance

    d. Drop the issue because non-compliance is always a problem

23. How do accreditation organizations such as the Joint Commission use the health record?

    a. To serve as a source for case study information

    b. To determine whether the documentation supports the provider's claim for reimbursement

    c. To provide healthcare services

    d. To determine whether standards of care are being met

24. Valley High, a skilled nursing facility, wants to become certified to take part in federal government reimbursement programs such as Medicare. What standards must the facility meet in order to become certified for these programs?

    a. Joint Commission Accreditation Standards

    b. Accreditation Association for Ambulatory Healthcare Standards

    c. Conditions of Participation

    d. Outcomes and Assessment Information Set

25. Before healthcare organizations can provide services, they usually must obtain _____ by government entities such as the state in which they are located.

    a. Accreditation

    b. Certification

    c. Licensure

    d. Permission

26. This document includes a microscopic description of tissue excised during surgery:

    a. Recovery room record

    b. Pathology report

    c. Operative report

    d. Discharge summary

27. A health record with deficiencies that is not complete within the timeframe specified in the medical staff rules and regulations is called a(n) _____.

    a. Suspended record

    b. Delinquent record

    c. Pending record

    d. Illegal record

28. Bob Smith was admitted to Mercy Hospital on June 21. The physical was completed on June 23. According to Joint commission standards, which statement applies to this situation?

    a. The record is not in compliance as the physical exam must be completed within 24 hours of admission.

    b. The record is not in compliance as the physical exam must be completed within 48 hours of admission.

    c. The record is in compliance as the physical examination must be completed within 48 hours.

    d. The record is in compliance because the physical examination was completed within 72 hours of admission.

29. According to the Joint Commission Accreditation Standards, which document must be placed in the patient's record before a surgical procedure may be performed?

    a. Admission record

    b. Physician's order

    c. Report of history and physical examination

    d. Discharge summary

30. Which of the following programs have been in place in hospitals for years and have been

required by the Medicare and Medicaid programs and accreditation standards?

    a. Internal DRG audits

    b. Peer review

    c. Managed care

    d. Quality improvement

31. The HIM director is having difficulty with the on-call physicians in the emergency services department completing their health records. Currently, three deficiency notices are sent to the physicians including an initial notice, a second reminder, and a final notification. Which of the following would be the best first step in trying to rectify the current situation?

    a. Routinely send out a fourth notice

    b. Post the hospital policy in the emergency department

    c. Consult with the physician in charge of the on-call doctors for suggestions on how to improve response to the current notices

    d. Call the Joint Commission

32. HIM coding professionals and the organizations that employ them have the responsibility to not tolerate behavior that adversely affects data quality. Which of the following is an example of behavior that should not be tolerated?

    a. Assign codes to an incomplete record with organizational policies in place to ensure codes are reviewed after the records are complete

    b. Follow up on and monitor identified problems

    c. Evaluate and trend diagnoses and procedures code selections

    d. Report data quality review results to organizational leadership, compliance staff, and the medical staff

33. What is the name of the formal document prepared by the surgeon at the conclusion of surgery to describe the surgical procedure performed?

    a. Operative report

    b. Tissue report

    c. Pathology report

    d. Anesthesia record

34. Where would information on treatment given on a particular encounter be found in the health record?

    a. Problem list

    b. Physician's orders

    c. Progress notes

    d. Physical examination

Domain 3: Clinical Classification Systems

35. Identify the code for a patient with a closed transcervical fracture of the epiphysis.

    a. 820.09

    b. 820.02

    c. 820.03

    d. 820.01

36. Identify the ICD-9-CM diagnosis code(s) for neonatal tooth eruption.

    a. 525.0

    b. 520.6, 525.0

    c. 520.9

    d. 520.6

37. Identify CPT code(s) for the following patient. A 35-year-old female undergoes an excision of a 3.0-cm tumor of her forehead. An incision is made through the skin and subcutaneous tissue. The tumor is dissected free of surrounding structures. The wound is closed in layers and interrupted sutures.

    a. 21012

    b. 21012; 12052

    c. 21014

    d. 21014; 12052

38. Identify CPT code(s) for the following Medicare patient. A 67-year-old female undergoes a fine needle aspiration of the left breast with ultrasound guidance to place a localization clip during a breast biopsy.

    a. 10022

    b. 10022; 19295–LT

    c. 10022; 19295–LT; 76942

    d. 10022; 76942

39. Identify the appropriate ICD-9-CM diagnosis code for Lou Gehrig's disease.

    a. 335.20

    b. 334.8

    c. 335.29

    d. 335.2

40. Identify the ICD-9-CM procedure code(s) for insertion of dual chamber cardiac pacemaker and atrial and ventricular leads.

    a. 37,83, 37.73

    b. 37.83, 37.71

    c. 37.81, 37.73, 37.71

    d. 37.83, 37.72

41. Identify the correct ICD-9-CM procedure code(s) for replacement of an old dual pacemaker with a new dual pacemaker.

    a. 37.87

    b. 37.85

    c. 37.87, 37.89

    d. 37.85, 37.89

42. Identify the appropriate ICD-9-CM diagnosis code(s) for right and left bundle branch block.

    a. 426.3, 426.4

    b. 426.53

    c. 426.4, 426.53

    d. 426.52

43. Identify the appropriate diagnostic and/or procedure ICD-9-CM code(s) for reprogramming of a cardiac pacemaker.

    a. V53.31

    b. 37.85

    c. V53.02

    d. V53.31, 37.85

44. This is a condition with an imprecise diagnosis with various characteristics. The condition may be diagnosed when a patient presents with sinus arrest, sinoatrial exit block, or persistent sinus bradycardia. This syndrome is often the result of drug therapy, such as digitalis, calcium channel blockers, beta-blockers, sympatholytic agents, or antiarrhythmics. Another presentation includes recurrent supraventricular tachycardias associated with brady-arrhythmias. Prolonged ambulatory monitoring may be indicated to establish a diagnosis of this condition. Treatment includes insertion of a permanent cardiac pacemaker.

    a. Atrial fibrillation (427.31)

    b. Atrial flutter (427.32)

    c. Paroxysmal supraventricular tachycardia (427.0)

    d. Sick sinus syndrome (SSS) (427.81)

45. Identify the appropriate ICD-9-CM procedure code(s) for a double internal mammary-coronary artery bypass.

    a. 36.15, 36.16

    b. 36.15

    c. 36.16

    d. 36.12, 36.16

46. Coronary arteriography serves as a diagnostic tool in detecting obstruction within the coronary arteries. Identify the technique using two catheters inserted percutaneously through the femoral artery.

    a. Combined right and left (88.54)

    b. Stones (88.55)

    c. Judkins (88.56)

    d. Other and unspecified (88.57)

47. Identify the correct diagnosis ICD-9-CM code(s) for a patient who arrives at the hospital for outpatient laboratory services ordered by the physician to monitor the patient's Coumadin levels. A prothrombin time (PT) is performed to check the patient's long-term use of his anticoagulant treatment.

    a. V58.83, V58.61

    b. V58.83, V58.63

    c. V58.61, 790.92

    d. V58.61

48. Identify the CPT code(s) for the following patient: A 2-year-old male presented to the emergency room in the middle of the night to have his nasogastric feeding tube repositioned through the duodenum under fluoroscopic guidance.

    a. 43752

    b. 43761

    c. 43761; 76000

    d. 49450

49. Identify the CPT code(s) for the following patient: A 2-year-old male presented to the hospital to have his gastrostomy tube changed under fluoroscopic guidance.

    a. 43752

    b. 43760

    c. 43761; 76000

    d. 49450

50. Identify the ICD-9-CM diagnosis code for blighted ovum.

    a. 236.1

    b. 661.00

    c. 631

    d. 634.90

51. Identify the ICD-9-CM diagnostic code(s) for the following: threatened abortion with hemorrhage at 15 weeks; home undelivered.

    a. 640.01, 640.91

    b. 640.03

    c. 640.83

    d. 640.80

52. Identify the ICD-9-CM diagnostic code(s) and procedure code(s) for the following: term pregnancy with failure of cervical dilation; lower uterine segment Cesarean delivery with single live-born female.

    a. 661.01, V27.0, 74.1

    b. 661.21, 74.1

    c. 661.01, 74.0

    d. 661.21, V27, 74.1

53. Identify the ICD-9-CM code for diaper rash, elderly patient.

    a. 690.10

    b. 691.0

    c. 782.1

    d. 705.1

54. Identify the ICD-9-CM code(s) for infected ingrown nail.

    a. 703.0

    b. 703.8, 681.11

    c. 681.11

    d. 681.9

55. Identify the ICD-9-CM code for acute lymphadenitis.

    a. 785.6

    b. 683

    c. 289.1

    d. 289.3

56. Identify the ICD-9-CM diagnostic code for primary localized osteoarthrosis of the hip.

    a. 715.95

    b. 715.15

    c. 721.90

    d. 715.16

57. Identify the ICD-9-CM diagnosis code for chondromalacia of the patella.

    a. 717.7

    b. 733.92

    c. 748.3

    d. 716.86

58. Identify the ICD-9-CM diagnosis code for Paget's disease of the bone (no bone tumor noted):

    a. 170.9

    b. 213.9

    c. 238.0

    d. 731.0

59. Identify the ICD-9-CM diagnostic code(s) for acute osteomyelitis of ankle due to staphylococcus.

    a. 730.06

    b. 730.07

    c. 730.07, 041.1

    d. 730.07, 041.10

60. Identify the ICD-9-CM diagnostic code for other specified aplastic anemia secondary to chemotherapy.

    a. 284.9

    b. 284.89

    c. 285.9

    d. 285.22

61. Identify the ICD-9-CM diagnostic code(s) for the following: A 6-month-old child is scheduled for a clinic visit for a routine well child exam. The physician documents, "well child, ex-preemie."

    a. V20.1, 765.10

    b. V20.2

    c. V20.2, 765.10

    d. V20.2, 765.19

62. Identify the ICD-9-CM diagnostic code for diastolic dysfunction.

    a. 428.1

    b. 428.30

    c. 428.9

    d. 429.9

63. Identify the ICD-9-CM procedure code(s) for the following: A 73-year-old female was treated for hemorrhage of the inferior mesenteric artery. She was admitted to the hospital for a transcatheter embolization of the bleeders with polyvinyl alcohol (PVA) microspheres and coils and abdominal angiography.

    a. 39.73, 88.47

    b. 39.71, 88.47

    c. 39.79, 88.49

    d. 39.79, 88.47

64. Identify ICD-9-CM procedure code for allogeneic donor lymphocyte stem cell infusion.

    a. 41.02

    b. 41.03

    c. 41.05

    d. 41.08

65. Identify ICD-9-CM diagnosis code for atypical ductal hyperplasia.

    a. 610.1

    b. 610.4

    c. 610.8

    d. 610.9

66. Which of the following is the correct ICD-9-CM procedure code for a Mayo operation known as a bunionectomy?

    a. 77.54

    b. 77.69

    c. 77.59

    d. 77.51

67. Which of the following is the correct ICD-9-CM code(s) for thoracoscopic lobectomy of left lung?

    a. 32.30

    b. 32.41

    c. 32.49

    d. 34.02, 32.41

68. Which of the following is the correct ICD-9-CM code(s) for laparoscopic cholecystectomy?

    a. 51.21

    b. 51.22, 54.21

    c. 51.23, 54.21

    d. 51.23

69. Which of the following is the correct ICD-9-CM procedure code(s) for cystoscopy with biopsy?

    a. 57.34

    b. 57.32, 57.33

    c. 57.33

    d. 57.39

70. Identify the ICD-9-CM procedure code(s) for insertion of tissue expander in breast, post mastectomy.

    a. 85.94

    b. 85.89

    c. 86.89, 85.46

    d. 85.95

Domain 4: Reimbursement Methodologies

71. Which of the following software applications would be used to aid in the coding function in a physician's office?

    a. Grouper

    b. Encoder

    c. Pricer

    d. Diagnosis calculator

72. Which payment system was introduced in 1992 and replaced Medicare's customary, prevailing, and reasonable (CPR) payment system?

    a. Diagnosis-related groups

    b. Resource-based relative value scale system

    c. Long-term care drugs

    d. Resource utilization groups

73. The patient had a total abdominal hysterectomy with bilateral salpingo-oophorectomy. The coder assigned the following codes:

    58150, Total abdominal hysterectomy, with/without removal of tubes and ovaries

    58700, Salpingectomy, complete or partial, unilateral/bilateral (separate procedure)

    What error has the coder made by using these codes?

    a. Maximizing

    b. Upcoding

    c. Unbundling

    d. Optimizing

74. What is the best reference tool to determine how CPT codes should be assigned?

    a. Local coverage determination from Medicare

    b. American Medical Association's CPT Assistant newsletter

    c. American Hospital Association's Coding Clinic

    d. CMS Web site

75. An electrolyte panel (80051) in the laboratory section of CPT consists of tests for carbon dioxide (82374), chloride (82435), potassium (84132), and sodium (84295). If each of the component codes are reported and billed individually on a claim form, this would be a form of:

    a. Optimizing

    b. Unbundling

    c. Sequencing

    d. Classifying

76. In the laboratory section of CPT, if a group of tests overlaps two or more panels, report the panel that incorporates the greater number of tests to fulfill the code definition. What would a coder do with the remaining test codes that are not part of a panel?

    a. Report the remaining tests using individual test codes according to CPT.

    b. Do not report the remaining individual test codes.

    c. Report only those test codes that are part of a panel.

    d. Do not report a test code more than once regardless if the test was performed twice.

77. There are several codes to describe a colonoscopy. CPT code 45378 describes the most basic colonoscopy without additional services. Additional codes in the colonoscopy section of CPT further define removal of foreign body (45379) and biopsy, single or multiple (45380) and others. Reporting the basic form of a colonoscopy (45378) with a foreign body (45379) or biopsy code (45380) would violate which rule?

    a. Unbundling

    b. Optimizing

    c. Sequencing

    d. Maximizing

78. What did the Centers of Medicare and Medicaid Services develop to promote national correct coding methodologies and to control improper coding leading to inappropriate payment in Part B claims?

    a. Outpatient Perspective Payment System (OPPS)

    b. National Correct Coding Initiative (NCCI)

    c. Ambulatory Payment Classifications (APCs)

    d. Comprehensive Outpatient Rehab Facilities (CORFs)

79. What is the best reference tool to receive ICD-9-CM coding advice?

    a. AMA's *CPT Assistant*

    b. AHA's *Coding Clinic for HCPCS*

    c. AHA's *Coding Clinic for ICD-9-CM*

    d. National Correct Coding Initiative (NCCI)

80. CMS developed Medically Unlikely Edits (MUEs) to prevent providers from billing units of services greater than the norm would indicate. These MUEs were implemented on January 1, 2007 and are applied to which code set?

    a. Diagnosis-related groups

    b. HCPCS/CPT codes

    c. ICD-9-CM diagnosis and procedure codes

    d. Resource utilization groups

Domain 5: Information and Communication Technologies

81. A hospital HIM department wants to purchase an electronic system that records the location of health records removed from the filing system and documents the date of their return to the HIM department. Which of the following electronic systems would fulfill this purpose?

    a. Chart deficiency system

    b. Chart tracking system

    c. Chart abstracting system

    d. Chart encoder

82. What does an audit trail check for?

    a. Unauthorized access to a system

    b. Loss of data

    c. Presence of a virus

    d. Successful completion of a backup

83. An individual designated as an inpatient coder may have access to an electronic medical record in order to code the record. Under what access security mechanism is the coder allowed access to the system?

    a. Role-based

    b. User-based

    c. Context-based

    d. Situation-based

84. Which of the following statements about a firewall is **false**?

    a. It is a system or combination of systems that supports an access control policy between two networks.

    b. The most common place to find a firewall is between the healthcare organization's internal network and the Internet.

    c. Firewalls are effective for preventing all types of attacks on a healthcare system.

    d. A firewall can limit internal users from accessing various portions of the Internet.

85. The technology commonly utilized for automated claims processing (sending bills directly to third-party payers) is _____.

    a. Optical character recognition

    b. Bar coding

    c. Neural networks

    d. Electronic data interchange

86. A software interface is a _____.

    a. Device to enter data

    b. Protocol for describing data

    c. Program to exchange data

    d. Standard vocabulary

Domain 6: Privacy, Confidentiality, Legal, and Ethical Issues

87. A hospital receives a valid request from a patient for copies of her medical records. The HIM clerk who is preparing the records removes copies of the patient's records from another hospital where the patient was previously treated. According to HIPAA regulations, was this action correct?

    a. Yes; HIPAA only requires that current records be produced for the patient.

    b. Yes; this is hospital policy for which HIPAA has no control.

    c. No; the records from the previous hospital are considered part of the designated record set and should be given to the patient.

    d. No; the records from the previous hospital are not included in the designated record set but should be released anyway.

88. A patient requests copies of her personal health information on CD. When the patient goes home, she finds that she cannot read the CD on her computer. The patient then requests the hospital provide the medical records in paper format. How should the hospital respond?

    a. Provide the medical records in paper format

    b. Burn another CD since this is hospital policy

    c. Provide the patient with both paper and CD copies of the medical record

    d. Review the CD copies with the patient on a hospital computer

89. Which of the following definitions **best** describes the concept of confidentiality?

    a. The right of individuals to control access to their personal health information

    b. The protection of healthcare information from damage, loss, and unauthorized alteration

    c. The expectation that personal information shared by an individual with a healthcare provider during the course of care will be used only for its intended purpose

    d. The expectation that only individuals with the appropriate authority will be allowed to access healthcare information

90. The release of information function requires the HIM professional to have knowledge of _____.

    a. Clinical coding principals

    b. Database development

    c. Federal and state confidentiality laws

    d. Human resource management

91. The Medical Record Committee is reviewing the privacy policies for a large outpatient clinic. One of the members of the committee remarks that he feels the clinic's practice of calling out a patient's full name in the waiting room is not in compliance with HIPAA regulations and that only the patient's first name should be used. Other committee members disagree with this assessment. What should the HIM director advise the committee?

    a. HIPAA does not allow a patient's name to be announced in a waiting room.

    b. There is no HIPAA violation for announcing a patient's name, but the committee may want to consider implementing practices that might reduce this practice.

    c. HIPAA allows only the use of the patient's first name.

    d. HIPAA requires that patients be given numbers and only the number be announced.

92. A health information technician receives a subpoena *duces tecum* for the records of a discharged patient. To respond to the subpoena, which of the following should the technician do?

    a. Review the subpoena to determine what documents must be produced

    b. Review the subpoena and notify the hospital administrator

    c. Consult with the hospital legal counsel

    d. Review the subpoena and alert the hospital risk-management department

93. The right of an individual to keep information about himself or herself from being disclosed to anyone is a definition of:

    a. Confidentiality

    b. Privacy

    c. Integrity

    d. Security

94. What types of covered entity health records are subject to HIPAA privacy regulations?

    a. Only health records in paper format

    b. Only health records in electronic format

    c. Health records in paper or electronic format

    d. Health records in any format

95. Mary Smith has gone to her doctor to discuss her current medical condition. What is the legal term that best describes the type of communication that has occurred between Mary and her physician?

    a. Closed communication

    b. Open communication

    c. Private communication

    d. Privileged communication

96. Dr. Smith, a member of the medical staff, asks to see the medical records of his adult daughter who was hospitalized in your institution for a tonsillectomy at age 16. The daughter is now 25. Dr. Jones was the patient's physician. Of the options listed here, what is the best course of action?

    a. Allow Dr. Smith to see the records because he was the daughter's guardian at the time of the tonsillectomy.

    b. Call the hospital administrator for authorization to release the record to Dr. Smith since he is on the medical staff.

    c. Inform Dr. Smith that he cannot access his daughter's health record without her signed authorization allowing him access to the record.

    d. Refer Dr. Smith to Dr. Jones and release the record if Dr. Jones agrees.

97. Which of the following four sources of law is also known as judge-made or case law?

    a. Constitutional law

    b. Statutory law

    c. Common law

    d. Administrative law

98. The sequence of the correct steps when evaluating an ethical problem is:

    a. Consider the values and obligations of others; consider the choices that are both justified and not justified; determine the facts; identify prevention options.

    b. Consider the choices that are both justified and not justified; consider the values and obligations of others; identify prevention options; determine the facts.

    c. Determine the facts; consider the choices that are both justified and not justified; consider the values and obligations of others; identify prevention options.

    d. Determine the facts; consider the values and obligations of others; consider the choices that are both justified and not justified; identify prevention options.

99. What should a hospital do when a state law requires more stringent privacy protection than the federal HIPAA privacy standard?

    a. Ignore the state law and follow the HIPAA standard

    b. Follow the state law and ignore the HIPAA standard

    c. Comply with both the state law and the HIPAA standard

    d. Ignore both the state law and the HIPAA standard and follow relevant accreditation standards

100. Jack Mitchell, a patient in Ross Hospital, is being treated for gallstones. He has not opted out of the facility directory. Callers who request information about him may be given:

    a. No information due to the highly sensitive nature of his illness

    b. Admission date and location in the facility

    c. General condition and acknowledgement of admission

    d. Location in the facility and diagnosis

Certified Coding Associate
Exam Preparation

Exam 2

Domain 1: Health Records and Data Content

1. Documentation regarding a patient's marital status, dietary, sleep, and exercise patterns, use of coffee, tobacco, alcohol, and other drugs may be found in the _____.

   a. Physical examination record

   b. History record

   c. Operative report

   d. Radiological report

2. A patient with known COPD and hypertension under treatment was admitted to the hospital with symptoms of a lower abdominal pain. He undergoes a laparoscopic appendectomy and develops a fever. The patient was subsequently discharged from the hospital with a principal diagnosis of acute appendicitis and secondary diagnoses of post-operative infection, COPD, and hypertension. Which of the following diagnoses should not be tagged as POA?

   a. Postoperative infection

   b. Appendicitis

   c. COPD

   d. Hypertension

3. Which of the following would **not** be found in a medical history?

   a. Chief complaint

   b. Vital signs

   c. Present illness

   d. Review of systems

4. Which of the following documentation must be included in a patient's medical record prior to performing a surgical procedure?

   a. Consent for operative procedure, anesthesia report, surgical report

   b. Consent for operative procedure, history, physical examination

   c. History, physical examination, anesthesia report

   d. Problem list, history, physical examination

5. Which of the following reports include names of the surgeon and assistants, date, duration, and description of the procedure and any specimens removed?

   a. Operative report

   b. Anesthesia report

   c. Pathology report

   d. Laboratory report

6. Identify the acute-care record report where the following information would be found: The patient is well-developed, obese male who does not appear to be in any distress, but has considerable problem with mobility. He has difficulty rising up from a chair and he uses a cane to ambulate. VITAL SIGNS: His blood pressure today is 158/86, pulse is 80 per minute, weight is 204 pounds (which is 13 pounds below what he weighed in April). He has no pallor. He has rather pronounced shaking of his arms, which he claims is not new. NECK: Showed no jugular venous distension. HEART: Very irregular. LUNGS: Clear. EXTREMITIES: Show edema of both legs.

   a. Discharge summary

   b. Medical history

   c. Medical laboratory report

   d. Physical examination

7. Identify the acute care record report where the following information would be found: Gross Description: Received fresh designated left lacrimal gland is a single, unoriented, irregular tan-pink portion of soft tissue measuring $0.8 \times 0.6 \times 0.1$ cm, which is submitted entirely, intact, in one cassette.

   a. Medical history

   b. Medical laboratory report

   c. Pathology report

   d. Physical examination

8. The clinical statement, "microscopic sections of the gallbladder reveals a surface lined by tall columnar cells of uniform size and shape" would be documented on which medical record form?

   a. Operative report

   b. Pathology report

   c. Discharge summary

   d. Nursing note

9. Both HEDIS and the Joint Commission's ORYX program are designed to collect data to be used for _____.

   a. Performance improvement programs

   b. Billing and claims data processing

   c. Developing hospital discharge abstracting systems

   d. Developing individual care plans for residents

10. What is abstracting?

    a. Compiling the pertinent information from the medical record based on predetermined data sets

    b. Assigning the appropriate code or nomenclature term for categorization

    c. Assembling a chronological set of data for an express purpose

    d. Conducting qualitative and quantitative analysis of documentation against standards and policy

11. What type of standard establishes uniform definitions for clinical terms?

    a. Identifier standard

    b. Vocabulary standard

    c. Transaction and messaging standard

    d. Structure and content standard

12. According to ICD-9-CM, an *elderly primigravida* is defined as a woman who gives birth to her first child at the age of _____ or older:

    a. 30

    b. 35

    c. 38

    d. 40

13. ICD-9-CM defines the "newborn period" as birth through the _____ day following birth.

    a. 28th

    b. 14th

    c. 60th

    d. 30th

14. "Late pregnancy" (category code 645) is used to demonstrate that a woman is over _____.

    a. 41

    b. 39

    c. 40

    d. 42

15. Which of the following would be classified to an ICD-9-CM category for bacterial diseases?

    a. Herpes simplex

    b. Staphylococcus aureus

    c. Influenza, types A and B

    d. Candida albicans

16. The coder notes that the physician has prescribed Retrovir for the patient. The coder might find which of the following on the patient's discharge summary?

    a. Otitis media

    b. AIDS

    c. Toxic shock syndrome

    d. Bacteremia

17. What diagnosis would the coder expect to see when a patient with pneumonia has inhaled food, liquid, or oil?

    a. Lobar pneumonia

    b. Pneumocystitis carinii pneumonia

    c. Interstitial pneumonia

    d. Aspiration pneumonia

18. Where would a coder who needed to locate the histology of a tissue sample most likely find this information?

    a. Pathology report

    b. Progress notes

    c. Nurse's notes

    d. Operative report

19. The coder notes the patient is taking prescribed Haldol. The final diagnoses on the progress notes include diabetes mellitus, acute pharyngitis, and malnutrition. What condition might the coder suspect the patient has and should query the physician?

    a. Insomnia

    b. Hypertension

    c. Schizophrenia

    d. Rheumatoid arthritis

Domain 2: Health Information Requirements and Standards

20. Which organization developed the first hospital standardization program?

    a. Joint Commission

    b. American Osteopathic Association

    c. American College of Surgeons

    d. American Association of Medical Colleges

21. The hospital is revising its policy on medical record documentation. Currently, all entries in the medical record must be legible, complete, dated, and signed. The committee chairperson wants to add that, in addition, all entries must have the time noted. However, another clinician suggests that adding the time of notation is difficult and rarely may be correct since personal watches and hospital clocks may not be coordinated. Another committee member agrees and says only electronic documentation needs a time stamp. Given this discussion, which of the following might the HIM director suggest?

    a. Suggest that only hospital clock time be noted in clinical documentation

    b. Suggest that only electronic documentation have time notated

    c. Inform the committee that according to the Medicare Conditions of Participation all documentation must be authenticated and dated

    d. Inform the committee that according to the Medicare Conditions of Participation only medication orders must include date and time

22. When correcting erroneous information in a health record, which of the following is **not** appropriate?

    a. Print "error" above the entry

    b. Enter the correction in chronological sequence

    c. Add the reason for the change

    d. Use black pen to obliterate the entry

23. Community Hospital implemented a clinical document improvement (CDI) program six months ago. The goal of the program was to improve clinical documentation to support quality of care, data quality, and HIM coding accuracy. Which of the following would be **best** to ensure that everyone understands the importance of this program?

    a. Request that the CEO write a memorandum to all hospital staff

    b. Give the chairperson of the CDI committee authority to fire employees who don't improve their clinical documentation

    c. Include ancillary clinical and medical staff in the process

    d. Request a letter from the Joint Commission

24. In a routine health record quantitative analysis review it was found that a physician dictated a discharge summary on 1/26/2009. The patient, however, was discharged two days later. In this case, what would be the best course of action?

    a. Request that the physician dictate another discharge summary

    b. Have the record analyst note the date discrepancy

    c. Request the physician dictate an addendum to the discharge summary

    d. File the record as complete since the discharge summary includes all of the pertinent patient information

25. During an audit of health records, the HIM director finds that transcribed reports are being changed by the author up to a week after initial transcription. The director is concerned that changes occurring this long after transcription jeopardize the legal principle that documentation must occur near the time of the event. To remedy this situation, the HIM director should recommend which of the following?

    a. Immediately stop the practice of changing transcribed reports

    b. Develop a facility policy that defines the acceptable period of time allowed for a transcribed document to remain in draft form

    c. Conduct a verification audit

    d. Alert hospital legal counsel of the practice

26. During a review of documentation practices, the HIM director finds that nurses are routinely using the copy and paste function of the hospital's new EHR system for documenting nursing notes. In some cases, nurses are copying and pasting the objective data from the lab system and intake-output records as well as the patient's subjective complaints and symptoms originally documented by another practitioner. Which of the following should the HIM director do to ensure the nurses are following acceptable documentation practices?

    a. Inform the nurses that "copy and paste" is not acceptable and to stop this practice immediately

    b. Determine how many nurses are involved in this practice

    c. Institute an in-service training session on documentation practices

    d. Develop policies and procedures related to cutting, copying, and pasting documentation in the EHR system

27. Who is responsible for writing and signing discharge summaries and discharge instructions?

    a. Attending physician

    b. Head nurse

    c. Primary physician

    d. Admitting nurse

28. Dr. Jones has signed a statement that all of her dictated reports should be automatically considered approved and signed unless she makes corrections within 72 hours of dictating. This is called _____.

    a. Autoauthentication

    b. Electronic signature

    c. Automatic record completion

    d. Chart tracking

29. The discharge summary must be completed within _____ after discharge for most patients but within _____ for patients transferred to other facilities. Discharge summaries are not always required for patients who were hospitalized for less than _____ hours.

    a. 30 days/48 hours/24 hours

    b. 14 days/24 hours/48 hours

    c. 14 days/48 hours/24 hours

    d. 30 days/24 hours/48 hours

30. Which of the following is **not** an accepted accrediting body for behavioral healthcare organizations?

    a. American Psychological Association

    b. Joint Commission

    c. Commission on Accreditation of Rehabilitation Facilities

    d. National Committee for Quality Assurance

31. What type of standard establishes methods for creating unique designations for individual patients, healthcare professionals, healthcare provider organizations, and healthcare vendors and suppliers?

    a. Vocabulary standard

    b. Identifier standard

    c. Structure and content standard

    d. Security standard

32. What type of organization works under contract with the CMS to conduct Medicare and Medicaid certification surveys for hospitals?

    a. Accreditation organizations

    b. Certification organizations

    c. State licensure agencies

    d. Conditions of participation agencies

33. Which of the following specialized patient assessment tools must be used by Medicare-certified home care providers?

    a. Patient Assessment Instrument

    b. Minimum Data Set for Long-Term Care

    c. Resident Assessment Protocol

    d. Outcomes and Assessment Information Set

Domain 3: Clinical Classification Systems

34. Identify the correct sequence and ICD-9-CM diagnosis code(s) for a patient with a scar on the right hand secondary to a laceration sustained two years ago.

    a. 709.2

    b. 906.1

    c. 709.2, 906.1

    d. 906.1, 709.2

35. Identify the correct sequence and ICD-9-CM diagnosis code(s) for a patient with dysphasia secondary to old cerebrovascular accident sustained one year ago.

    a. 787.20, 438.12

    b. 784.59, 438.12

    c. 438.12

    d. 787.20, 438.89

36. Identify the correct ICD-9-CM diagnosis code(s) for a patient with nausea, vomiting, and gastroenteritis.

    a. 558.9

    b. 787.01, 558.9

    c. 787.02, 787.03, 558.9

    d. 787.01, 558.41

37. Identify the correct ICD-9-CM diagnosis code for a patient with an elevated prostate specific antigen (PSA) test result.

    a. 796.4

    b. 790.6

    c. 792.9

    d. 790.93

38. Identify the correct ICD-9-CM diagnosis code(s) for a patient with near-syncope event and nausea.

    a. 780.2

    b. 780.2, 787.02

    c. 780.2, 787.01

    d. 780.4, 787.02

39. Identify the correct ICD-9-CM diagnosis code(s) for a patient with abnormal glucose tolerance test.

    a. 790.29

    b. 790.21

    c. 790.21, 790.29

    d. 790.22

40. Identify the correct ICD-9-CM diagnosis code(s) for a patient with pneumonia and persistent cough.

    a. 786.2, 490

    b. 486, 786.2

    c. 486

    d. 481

41. Identify the correct ICD-9-CM diagnosis code(s) for a patient with seizures; epilepsy, ruled out.

    a. 780.39

    b. 345.9

    c. 780.39, 345.9

    d. 345.90

42. Identify the correct ICD-9-CM diagnosis code for a male patient with stress urinary incontinence.

    a. 625.6

    b. 788.30

    c. 788.32

    d. 788.39

43. Identify the correct ICD-9-CM diagnosis code(s) for a patient with right lower quadrant abdominal pain with nausea, vomiting, and diarrhea.

    a. 789.03

    b. 789.03, 787.02, 787.03, 787.91

    c. 789.03, 787.91

    d. 789.03, 787.01, 787.91

44. Identify the punctuation mark that is used to supplement words or explanatory information that may or may not be present in the statement of a diagnosis or procedure in ICD-9-CM coding. The punctuation does not affect the code number assigned to the case. The punctuation is considered a nonessential modifier, and all three volumes of ICD-9-CM use them.

    a. Parentheses ( )

    b. Square brackets [ ]

    c. Slanted brackets *[ ]*

    d. Braces { }

45. From the health record of a patient newly diagnosed with a malignancy:

> **Preoperative Diagnosis:** Suspicious lesions, main bronchus
>
> **Postoperative Diagnosis:** Carcinoma, in situ, main bronchus
>
> **Indications:** Previous bronchoscopy showed two suspicious lesions in the main bronchus. Laser photoresection is planned for destruction of these lesions, because bronchial washings obtained previously showed carcinoma in situ.
>
> **Procedure:** Following general anesthesia in the hospital same-day surgery area, with a high-frequency jet ventilator, a rigid bronchoscope is inserted and advanced through the larynx to the main bronchus. The areas were treated with laser photoresection.

Identify the ICD-9-CM diagnosis code and CPT procedure code(s) for this service?

    a. 162.2, 31641, 31623–59

    b. 231.2, 31641, 31623–59

    c. 231.2, 31641

    d. 162.2, 31641

46. A 22-year-old patient presents for a closure of a patent ductus arteriosus. The patient's thorax is opened posteriorly and the vagus nerve is isolated away. The PDA is divided and sutured individually in the aorta and pulmonary artery. How is this procedure coded?

    a. 33813

    b. 33820

    c. 33822

    d. 33824

47. Identify the correct ICD-9-CM diagnosis code for a patient with anterolateral wall myocardial infarction, initial episode.

    a. 410.11

    b. 410.01

    c. 410.02

    d. 410.12

48. Identify the correct ICD-9-CM diagnosis code(s) and sequence for a patient with disseminated candidiasis secondary to AIDS-like syndrome.

    a. 042, 112.4, V01.79

    b. 112.4, 042

    c. 042, 112.4, V08

    d. 042, 112.4

49. Identify the correct ICD-9-CM diagnosis code(s) and proper sequencing for urinary tract infection due to *E. coli*.

    a. 599.0

    b. 599.0, 041.4

    c. 041.4

    d. 041.4, 599.0

50. Identify the correct ICD-9-CM diagnosis codes and sequence for a patient who was admitted to the outpatient chemotherapy floor for acute lymphocytic leukemia. During the procedure, the patient developed severe nausea with vomiting and was treated with medications.

    a. 204.00, 787.01, V58.11

    b. V58.11, 204.00, 787.01

    c. V58.11, 204.00

    d. 204.22, 787.01

51. Identify the correct ICD-9-CM diagnosis codes for metastatic carcinoma of the colon to the lung.

    a. 153.9, 162.9

    b. 197.0, 153.9

    c. 153.9, 197.0

    d. 153.9, 239.1

52. Identify the correct ICD-9-CM diagnosis code(s) for a patient with sepsis due to staphylococcus aureus septicemia.

    a. 038.11, 995.91

    b. 995.91, 038.11

    c. 038.11

    d. 038.11, 995.92

53. Identify the ICD-9-CM diagnosis code(s) for uncontrolled type II diabetes mellitus; mild malnutrition.

    a. 250.02

    b. 250.01, 263.1

    c. 250.02, 263.1

    d. 250.01, 263.0

54. Identify the ICD-9-CM diagnosis code(s) for neutropenic fever.

    a. 288.00

    b. 288.00, 780.60

    c. 288.01

    d. 288.00, 780.61

55. Identify the correct ICD-9-CM diagnosis code(s) for a patient who presents to the hospital outpatient department for a routine chest x-ray without signs and symptoms.

    a. V72.81

    b. V72.5

    c. V72.5, 793.99

    d. V70.9, 793.1

56. Mr. Smith is seen in his primary care physician's office for his annual physical examination. He has a digital rectal examination and is given three small cards to take home and return with fecal samples to screen for colorectal cancer. Assign the appropriate CPT code to report this occult blood sampling.

    a. 82270

    b. 82271

    c. 82272

    d. 82274

57. Category II codes cover all but one of the following topics. Which is **not** addressed by Category II codes?

    a. Patient management

    b. New technology

    c. Therapeutic, preventative, or other interventions

    d. Patient safety

58. Referencing the CPT codebook, a list of codes describing procedures that include conscious sedation, if administered by the same surgeon as performs the procedure, can be found in:

    a. Appendix E

    b. Appendix F

    c. Appendix G

    d. Appendix H

59. Per CPT guidelines, a separate procedure is:

    a. Coded when it is performed as part of another, larger procedure

    b. Considered to be an integral part of another, larger service

    c. Never coded under any circumstance

    d. Both a and b

60. CPT was developed and is maintained by:

    a. CMS

    b. AMA

    c. Cooperating Parties

    d. WHO

61. The codes in the musculoskeletal section of CPT may be used by:

    a. Orthopedic surgeons only

    b. Orthopedic surgeons and emergency department physicians

    c. Any physician

    d. Orthopedic surgeons and neurosurgeons

62. Observation E/M codes (99218 through 99220) are used in physician billing when:

    a. A patient is admitted and discharged on the same date.

    b. A patient is admitted for routine nursing care following surgery.

    c. A patient does not meet admission criteria.

    d. A patient is referred to a designated observation service.

63. Documentation in the history of use of drugs, alcohol, and/or tobacco is considered part of the:

    a. Past medical history

    b. Social history

    c. Systems review

    d. History of present illness

64. Tissue transplanted from one individual to another of the same species but different genotype is called a(n):

    a. Autograft

    b. Xenograft

    c. Allograft or allogeneic graft

    d. Heterograft

65. Mohs micrographic surgery involves the surgeon acting as:

    a. Both plastic surgeon and general surgeon

    b. Both surgeon and pathologist

    c. Both plastic surgeon and dermatologist

    d. Both dermatologist and pathologist

66. If an orthopedic surgeon attempted to reduce a fracture but was unsuccessful in obtaining acceptable alignment, what type of code should be assigned for the procedure?

    a. A "with manipulation" code

    b. A "without manipulation" code

    c. An unlisted procedure code

    d. An E/M code only

67. Identify the correct CPT procedure code for incision and drainage of infected shoulder bursa.

    a. 10060

    b. 10140

    c. 23030

    d. 23031

68. In coding arterial catheterizations, when the tip of the catheter is manipulated from the insertion into the aorta and then out into another artery, this is called:

    a. Selective catheterization

    b. Nonselective catheterization

    c. Manipulative catheterization

    d. Radical catheterization

69. When coding a selective catheterization in CPT, how are codes assigned?

    a. One code for each vessel entered

    b. One code for the point of entry vessel

    c. One code for the final vessel entered

    d. One code for the vessel of entry and one for the final vessel, with intervening vessels not coded

Domain 4: Reimbursement Methodologies

70. How does Medicare or other third-party payers determine whether the patient has medical necessity for the tests, procedures, or treatment billed on a claim form?

    a. By requesting the medical record for each service provided

    b. By reviewing all the diagnosis codes assigned to explain the reasons the services were provided

    c. By reviewing all physician orders

    d. By reviewing the discharge summary and history and physical for the patient over the last year

71. What is the name of the organization that develops the billing form that hospitals are required to use?

    a. American Academy of Billing Forms (AABF)

    b. National Uniform Billing Committee (NUBC)

    c. National Uniform Claims Committee (NUCC)

    d. American Billing and Claims Academy (ABCA)

72. What healthcare organizations collects UHDDS data?

    a. All outpatient settings including physician clinics and ambulatory surgical centers

    b. All outpatient settings including cancer centers, independent testing facilities, and nursing homes

    c. All non-outpatient settings including acute care, short term care, long term care, and psychiatric hospitals, home health agencies, rehabilitation facilities, and nursing homes

    d. All inpatient settings and outpatient settings with a focus on ambulatory surgical centers

73. What was the goal of the new MS-DRG system?

    a. To improve Medicare's capability to recognize severity of illness in its inpatient hospital payments. The new system is projected to increase payments to hospitals for services provided to sicker patients and decrease payments for treating less severely ill patients.

    b. To improve Medicare's capability to recognize poor quality of care and pay hospitals on an incentive grid that allows hospitals to be paid by performance.

    c. To improve Medicare's capability to recognize groups of data by patient populations which will further allow Medicare to adjust the hospitals wage indexes based on the data. This adjustment will be a system to pay hospitals fairly across all geographic locations.

    d. To improve Medicare's capability to recognize practice patterns among hospitals that are inappropriately optimizing payments by keeping patients in the hospital longer than the median length of stay.

74. What is the basic formula for calculating each MS-DRG hospital payment?

    a. Hospital payment = DRG relative weight × hospital base rate

    b. Hospital payment = DRG relative weight × hospital base rate − 1

    c. Hospital payment = DRG relative weight / hospital base rate + 1

    d. Hospital payment = DRG relative weight / hospital base rate

75. What are possible "add-on" payments that a hospital could receive in addition to the basic Medicare DRG payment?

    a. Additional payments may be made to locum tenens, increased emergency room services, stays over the average length of stay, and for cost outlier cases.

    b. Additional payments may be made to critical access hospitals, higher than normal volumes, unexpected hospital emergencies, and for cost outlier cases.

    c. Additional payments may be made to increased emergency room services, critical access hospitals, for increased labor costs, and for cost outlier cases.

    d. Additional payments may be made to disproportionate share hospitals, for indirect medical education, for new technologies, and for cost outlier cases.

76. What is the name of the national program to detect and correct improper payments in the Medicare Fee-for-Service (FFS) program?

    a. Medicare administrative contractors (MACs)

    b. Recovery audit contractors (RACs)

    c. Comprehensive error rate testing (CERT)

    d. Fiscal intermediaries (FIs)

77. What is the maximum number of procedure codes that can appear on a UB-04 paper claim form for a hospital inpatient?

    a. Three

    b. Nine

    c. Five

    d. Six

78. Which answer below is **not** correct for assignment of the MS-DRG?

    a. Diagnoses and procedures (principal and secondary)

    b. Attending and consulting physicians

    c. Presence of major or other complications and co morbidities (MCC or CC)

    d. Discharge disposition or status

79. What is the maximum number of diagnosis codes that can appear on the UB-04 paper claim form locator 67 for a hospital inpatient principle and secondary diagnoses?

    a. 22

    b. 18

    c. 16

    d. 9

Domain 5: Information and Communication Technologies

80. A hospital is planning on allowing coding professionals to work at home. The hospital is in the process of identifying strategies to minimize the security risks associated with this practice. Which of the following would be **best** to ensure that data breaches are minimized when the home computer is unattended?

    a. User name and password

    b. Automatic session terminations

    c. Cable locks

    d. Encryption

81. A coding analyst consistently enters the wrong code for patient gender in the electronic billing system. What security measures should be in place to minimize this security breach?

    a. Access controls

    b. Audit trail

    c. Edit checks

    d. Password controls

82. Which of the following would be the best technique to ensure that registration clerks consistently use the correct notation for assigning admission date in an electronic health record (EHR)?

    a. Make admission date a required field

    b. Provide an input mask for entering data in the field

    c. Make admission date a numeric field

    d. Provide sufficient space for input of data

83. In hospitals, automated systems for registering patients and tracking their encounters are commonly known as _____ systems.

    a. MIS

    b. CDS

    c. ADT

    d. ABC

84. Which of the following provides organizations with the ability to access data from multiple databases and to combine the results into a single questions-and-reporting interface?

    a. Client-server computer

    b. Data warehouse

    c. Local area network

    d. Internet

85. The _____ is a type of coding that is a natural outgrowth of the electronic health record.

    a. Automated codebook

    b. Computer-assisted coding

    c. Logic based encoder

    d. Decision support database

Domain 6: Privacy, Confidentiality, Legal, and Ethical Issues

86. A child was examined and treated for child abuse in the emergency department at the hospital. As a result, the child has been taken into protective custody by the Office of Child Protection because of suspected child abuse by the parents. The father requests copies of the designated record set for the visit. He has a copy of the child's birth certificate listing him as the father and he possesses a picture ID. Do you release a copy of the emergency department record?

    a. Yes, after he has completed a legitimate release of information authorization.

    b. Decline to release the information and contact the hospital's attorney.

    c. Contact the Office of Child Protection for permission to release the record.

    d. Refer the matter to the hospital administrator and follow the administration's instructions after he meets with the father.

87. A hospital currently includes the patient's social security number on the face sheet of the paper medical record and in the electronic version of the record. The hospital risk manager has identified this as a potential identity fraud risk and wants the information removed. The risk manager is not getting cooperation from the physicians and others in the hospital who say that they need the information for identification and other purposes. Given this situation, what should the HIM director suggest?

    a. Avoid displaying the number on any document, screen, or data collection field

    b. Allow the information in both electronic and paper forms since a variety of people need this data

    c. Require employees to sign confidentiality agreements if they have access to social security numbers

    d. Contact legal counsel for advice

88. Which of the following activities is considered an unethical practice?

    a. Backdating progress notes

    b. Performing quantitative analysis

    c. Verifying that an insurance company is one that is authorized to receive patient information

    d. Determining what information is required to fulfill an authorized request for information

89. Which of the following ethical principles is being followed when an HIT professional ensures that patient information is only released to those who have a legal right to access it?

    a. Autonomy

    b. Beneficence

    c. Justice

    d. Nonmaleficence

90. Although the HIPAA Privacy Rule allows patient access to personal health information about themselves, which of the following cannot be disclosed to patients?

    a. Interpretation of x-rays by the radiologist

    b. Billing records

    c. Progress notes written by the attending physician

    d. Psychotherapy notes

91. Which of the following is a core ethical obligation of health information staff?

    a. Coding diseases and operations

    b. Protecting patients' privacy and confidential communications

    c. Transcribing medical reports

    d. Performing quantitative analysis on record content

92. Under the HIPAA privacy standard, which of the following types of protected health information (PHI) must be specifically identified in an authorization?

    a. History and physical reports

    b. Operative reports

    c. Consultation reports

    d. Psychotherapy notes

93. What penalties can be enforced against a person or entity that willfully and knowingly violates the HIPAA Privacy Rule with the intent to sell, transfer, or use PHI for commercial advantage, personal gain, or malicious harm?

    a. A fine of not more than $10,000 only

    b. A fine of not more than $10,000, not more than 1 year in jail, or both

    c. A fine of not more than $5,000 only

    d. A fine of not more than $250,000, not more than 10 years in jail, or both

94. Today, Janet Kim visited her new dentist for an appointment. She was not presented with a Notice of Privacy Practices. Is this acceptable?

    a. No; a dentist is a healthcare clearinghouse, which is a covered entity under HIPAA.

    b. Yes; a dentist is not a covered entity per the HIPAA Privacy Rule.

    c. No; it is a violation of the HIPAA Privacy Rule.

    d. Yes; the Notice of Privacy Practices it not required until June 2012.

95. Mercy Hospital personnel need to review the medical records of Katie Grace for utilization review purposes (1). They will also be sending her records to her physician for continuity of care (2). Under HIPAA, these two functions are:

    a. Use (1) and disclosure (2)

    b. Request (1) and disclosure (2)

    c. Disclosure (1) and use (2)

    d. Disclosures (1 and 2)

96. Per the HIPAA Privacy Rule, which of the following requires authorization for research purposes?

    a. Use of Mary's information about her myocardial infarction, deidentified

    b. Use of Mary's information about her asthma, in a limited data set

    c. Use of Mary's individually identifiable information related to her asthma treatments

    d. Use of medical information about Jim, Mary's deceased husband

97. Which of the following activities would be in violation of AHIMA's Code of Ethics?

    a. Coding an intentionally inappropriate level of service

    b. Following established coding policies and procedures

    c. Protecting the confidentiality of patients' written and electronic records

    d. Taking remedial action when there is direct knowledge of a colleague's incompetence or impairment

98. An employee in the physical therapy department arrives early every morning to snoop through the clinical information system for potential information about neighbors and friends. What security mechanisms should be implemented to prevent this security breach?

    a. Audit controls

    b. Information access controls

    c. Facility access controls

    d. Workstation security

99. On review of the audit trail for an EHR system, the HIM director discovers that a departmental employee who has authorized access to patient records is printing far more records than the average user. In this case, what should the supervisor do?

    a. Reprimand the employee

    b. Fire the employee

    c. Determine what information was printed and why

    d. Revoke the employee's access privileges

100. What should a hospital do when a state law requires more stringent privacy protection than the federal HIPAA privacy standard?

   a. Ignore the state law and follow the HIPAA standard

   b. Follow the state law and ignore the HIPAA standard

   c. Comply with both the state law and the HIPAA standard

   d. Ignore both the state law and the HIPAA standard and follow relevant accreditation standards

Certified Coding Associate
Exam Preparation

Answer Key
Practice Answers

Domain 1

1. c (Johns 2007, chapter 2)

2. d Data quality includes these characteristics: accuracy, accessibility, comprehensiveness, consistency, currency, definition, granularity, precision, relevancy, and timeliness (Johns 2007, chapter 2).

3. c The operative report includes a description of the procedure performed (Johns 2007, chapter 3).

4. a Results for lab tests will be included in a medical laboratory report (Johns 2007, chapter 3).

5. d Results of an x-ray interpretation by a radiologist are reported in a radiography report (Johns 2007, chapter 3).

6. c Results of the physician's examination of the patient's physical condition is reported in a physical examination report (Johns 2007, chapter 3).

7. b Pathological examinations of tissue samples and tissues or organs removed during surgical procedures are reported in the pathology report (Johns 2007, chapter 3).

8. a (Johns 2007, chapter 3)

9. c This information is collected by the examination of a newborn and reported on the newborn record (Johns 2007, chapter 3).

10. c An ECG is a report of an electrocardiogram of the heart (Johns 2007, chapter 3).

11. b A consultation report includes the recommendations of a consulting physician who is requested to evaluate a patient (Johns 2007, chapter 3).

12. d (Johns 2007, chapter 3)

13. c Haldol may be used to treat mental or behavioral problems (http://www.drugs.com/pdr/haldol.html).

14. b Aspiration pneumonia results when a patient has inhaled body secretions, food, vomitus, or substances that are harmful or toxic when inhaled (Merck 2008c).

15. b If at the time of code assignment the documentation is unclear as to whether a condition was present on admission, it is appropriate to query the provider for clarification (CMS 2010c).

16. a In 1974, the federal government adopted the UHDDS as the standard for collecting data for the Medicare and Medicaid programs. When the Prospective Payment Act was enacted in 1983, UHDDS definitions were incorporated into the rules and regulations for implementing diagnosis-related groups (DRGs). A key component was the incorporation of the definitions of principal diagnosis, principal procedure, and other significant procedures, into the DRG algorithms (LaTour and Eichenwald Maki 2010, 165).

17. a (Johns 2007, chapter 5)

18. b (Johns 2007, chapter 5)

19. c (CMS 2010c)

20. a Subjective information includes symptoms and actions reported by the patient and not observed or measured by the healthcare provider (Johns 2007, chapter 3).

21. b Objective information may be measured or observed by the healthcare provider (Johns 2007, chapter 3).

22. d (Johns 2007, chapter 3)

23. c (Johns 2007, chapter 3)

24. d (Johns 2007, chapter 6)

25. b (Johns 2007, chapter 6)

26. c Data currency and data timeliness refer to the requirement that healthcare data should be up-to-date and recorded at or near the time of the event or observation (Johns 2007, chapter 2).

27. b Consistent data will be the same each time it is reported or collected (Johns 2007, chapter 2).

28. b (Johns 2007, chapter 2)

29. a (Johns 2007, chapter 3)

30. a (Johns 2007, chapter 3)

31. c (Johns 2007, chapter 3)

32. d (Johns 2007, chapter 3)

33. b (Johns 2007, chapter 3)

34. b (Johns 2007, chapter 3)

35. d (Johns 2007, chapter 2)

36. b (Johns 2007, chapter 3)

37. a (Johns 2007, chapter 3)

38. b (Johns 2007, chapter 3)

39. c (Johns 2007, chapter 3)

40. a *Hospice care* is palliative care provided to terminally ill patients and supportive services to patients and their families (Johns 2007, chapter 3).

Domain 2

41. c (Johns 2007, chapter 2)

42. b (Johns 2007, chapter 3)

43. b (Johns 2007, chapter 3)

44. a (Johns 2007, chapter 8)

45. c (Johns 2007, chapter 2)

46. a (Johns 2007, chapter 2)

47. b (Johns 2007, chapter 2)

48. b (Johns 2007, chapter 5)

49. c (Johns 2007, chapter 5)

50. a (Johns 2007, chapter 5)

51. c (Johns 2007, chapter 8)

52. d (Johns 2007, chapter 6)

53. d (Johns 2007, chapter 7)

54. a (Johns 2007, chapter 6)

55. b (Johns 2007, chapter 6)

56. c (Johns 2007, chapter 7)

57. b (Johns 2007, chapter 7)

58. d (Johns 2007, chapter 7)

59. d (Johns 2007, chapter 7)

60. c (Johns 2007, chapter 20)

61. d (Russo 2010, chapter 4)

62. b Concurrent review occurs on a continuing basis during a patient's stay (Johns 2007, chapter 20).

63. b Medicare required that all inpatient hospitals collect a minimum set of patient-specific data elements. These elements are in databases formulated from hospital discharge abstract systems. The patient specific data elements are referred to as the UHDDS (LaTour and Eichenwald Maki 2010, 165).

64. a Deemed status means accrediting bodies such as the Joint Commission or AOA can survey facilities for compliance with the Medicare Conditions of Participation for hospitals instead of government (Odom-Wesley et al. 2009, 291).

65. a The Medicare Conditions of Participation (2006) require that the patient's principal diagnosis be documented by the attending physician in the patient's health record no more than thirty days after discharge (Odom-Wesley et al. 2009, 201).

66. a *Qualitative analysis* is a review of the health record to ensure clinical protocols are met and determine the adequacy of entries documenting the quality of care (Odom-Wesley et al. 2009, 248).

67. b Long-term, acute-care hospitals are required to have physician acknowledgement statements signed and dated from the attending physician at the initial time of credentialing for admitting privileges just as is required for short-term acute-care hospitals (Odom-Wesley et al. 2009, 351).

68. a Adoption of the Minimum Standards was the basis of the Hospital Standardization Program and marked the beginning of the modern accreditation process for healthcare organizations. Basically, accreditation standards are developed to reflect reasonable quality standards (LaTour and Eichenwald Maki 2010, 11).

Domain 3

69. a Index Carcinoma, in situ, see also Neoplasm, by site, in situ (Schraffenberger 2010, 77–86).

70. b Index Melanoma (malignant), shoulder. Melanoma is considered a malignant neoplasm and is referenced as such in the index of ICD-9-CM. The term benign neoplasm is considered a growth that does not invade adjacent structures or spread to distant sites but may displace or exert pressure on adjacent structures (Schraffenberger 2010, 79, 83–84).

71. b (Johns 2007, chapter 6)

72. d (Johns 2007, chapter 6)

73. d (Johns 2007, chapter 6)

74. c (Johns 2007, chapter 6)

75. d (Johns 2007, chapter 6)

76. b (Johns 2007, chapter 6)

77. c (Johns 2007, chapter 6)

78. c Index Lipoma, face. ICD-9-CM classifies neoplasms by system, organ, or site with the exception of neoplasms of the lymphatic and hematopoietic system, malignant melanomas of the skin, lipomas, common tumors of the bone, uterus, and ovary. Because of these exceptions, the Alphabetic Index must first be checked to determine if a code has been assigned for that specific histology type (Schraffenberger, 77–86).

79. a Index Adenoma, adrenal (cortex). Index Syndrome, Conn. According to the index in ICD-9-CM, except where otherwise indicated, the morphological varieties of adenoma should be coded by site as for "Neoplasm, benign" (Schraffenberger 2010, 83–85).

80. a (Johns 2007, chapter 6)

81. c Index Contusion, cerebral—see Contusion, brain. Add a fifth digit of "2" for brief loss of consciousness. Cerebral contusions are often caused by a blow to the head. A cerebral contusion is a more severe injury involving a bruise of the brain with bleeding into the brain tissue, but without disruption of the brain's continuity. The loss of consciousness that occurs often lasts longer than that of a concussion. Codes for cerebral laceration and contusion range from 851.0–851.9, with fifth digits added to indicate whether a loss of consciousness or concussion occurred (Schraffenberger 2010, 271).

82. d The code selection is determined by measuring the greatest clinical diameter of the apparent lesion plus that margin required for complete excision (lesion diameter plus the most narrow margins required equals the excised diameter) (AMA 2010b, 60).

83. a Complex closure includes the repair of wounds requiring more than layered closure, viz., scar revision, débridement, extensive undermining, stents or retention sutures (AMA 2010b, 64).

84. d Signs and symptoms that are associated routinely with a disease process should not be assigned as additional codes, unless otherwise instructed by the classification (CMS 2010c, 10).

85. a Subsequent admissions for retained products of conception following a spontaneous or legally induced abortion are assigned the appropriate code from category 634, Spontaneous abortion, or 635 Legally induced abortion, with a fifth digit of "1" (incomplete). This advice is appropriate even when the patient was discharged previously with a discharge diagnosis of complete abortion (CMS 2010c, 50)

86. c The term *urosepsis* is a nonspecific term. If that is the only term documented, only code 599.0 should be assigned based on the default for the term in the ICD-9-CM index, in addition to the code for the causal organism, if known. Septicemia results from the entry of pathogens into the bloodstream. Symptoms include spiking fever, chills, and skin eruptions in the form of petichiae or purpura. Blood cultures are usually positive; however, a negative culture does not exclude the diagnosis of septicemia. Several other clinical indications and symptomology could indicate the diagnosis of septicemia. Only the physician can diagnose the condition based on clinical indications. Query the physician when the diagnosis is not clear to the coder (Schraffenberger 2010, 67–70; CMS 2010c, 18).

87. c If treatment is directed at the malignancy, designate the malignancy as the principal diagnosis. The only exception to this guideline is if a patient admission/encounter is solely for the administration of chemotherapy, immunotherapy, or radiation therapy, assign the appropriate V code as the first-listed or principal diagnosis and the diagnosis or problem for which the service is being performed as a secondary diagnosis (Schraffenberger 2010, 81–95; CMS 2010c, 25).

88. b Gastroenteritis is characterized by diarrhea, nausea, and vomiting, and abdominal cramps. Codes for symptoms, signs, and ill-defined conditions from Chapter 16 of the CPT codebook are not to be used as the principal diagnosis when a related definitive diagnosis has been established. Patients can have several chronic conditions that coexist at the time of their hospital admission and quality as additional diagnosis such as COPD and angina (Schraffenberger 2010, 51, 55, 184).

89. c When a primary malignancy has been previously excised or eradicated from its site and there is no further treatment directed to that site and there is no evidence of any existing primary malignancy, a code from category V10, Personal history of malignant neoplasm, should be used to indicate the former site of the malignancy. Any mention of extension, invasion, or metastatic to another site is coded as a secondary malignant neoplasm to that site. The secondary site may be the principal with the V10 code used as a secondary code (CMS 2010c, 25).

90. a In the unusual instance when two or more diagnoses equally meet the criteria for principal diagnosis, as determined by the circumstances of admission, diagnostic workup, and/or the therapy provided, and the Alphabetic Index, Tabular List, or another coding guideline does not provide sequencing direction in such cases, any one of the diagnoses may be sequenced first (Schraffenberger 2010, 52).

91. c For reporting purposes the definition for "other diagnoses" is interpreted as additional conditions that affect patient care in terms of requiring: clinical evaluation, therapeutic treatment, diagnostic procedures, extended length of hospital stay, increased nursing care, and/or monitoring (CMS 2010c, Section III, 93).

92. c A patient in status asthmaticus fails to respond to therapy administered during an asthmatic attack. This is a life-threatening condition that requires emergency care and likely hospitalization (Schraffenberger 2010, 173).

93. c Index Destruction, intervertebral disc, by other specified method

94. d Signs, symptoms, abnormal test results, or other reasons for the outpatient visit are used when a physician qualifies a diagnostic statement as "rule out" or other similar terms indicating uncertainty. In the outpatient setting the condition qualified in that statement should not be coded as if it existed. Rather, the condition should be coded to the highest degree of certainty, such as the sign or symptom the patient exhibits. In this case, assign the code 786.50, Chest pain NOS (Schraffenberger 2010, 259).

95. c For outpatient encounters for diagnostic tests that have been interpreted by a physician, and the final report is available at the time of coding, code any confirmed or definitive diagnosis(es) documented in the interpretation. Do not code related signs and symptoms as additional diagnosis. Note: This differs from the coding practice in the hospital inpatient setting regarding abnormal findings on test results (Schraffenberger 2010, 600).

96. c The disproportion was specified as cephalopelvic; thus the correct ICD-9-CM code is 653.41. Two codes are required for anesthesia; one for the planned vaginal delivery (01967) and an add-on code (01968) to describe anesthesia for Cesarean delivery following planned vaginal delivery converted to Cesarean. An instructional note guides the coder to use 01968 with 01967 (Schraffenberger 2010, 672; AMA 2010b, 48).

97. c   Code 99304 reports initial evaluation and management services to a nursing home patient. Code 99308 reports subsequent evaluation and management services that are performed to assess a change in the patient. Code 99306 reports an initial new or established nursing facility evaluation meeting comprehensive history, comprehensive exam, and high complexity medical decision making. Code 99318 is the appropriate code for an annual physical examination for administrative purposes (AHIMA 2010a, 679).

98. d   Code 45384 describes biopsy using a hot biopsy forceps. In addition, code 45342 is used to report a sigmoidoscopic ultrasound. Code 45391does not include the transmural biopsy that was performed via the ultrasonic endoscope (AHIMA 2010a, 653).

99. d   (Johns 2007, chapter 6)

100. d   (Johns 2007, chapter 6)

101. a   (Johns 2007, chapter 6)

102. a   Follow instructions under the main term in the Alphabetic Index. Instructions in the index should be followed when determining which column to use in the neoplasm table. In this example malignant is not a choice in the Alphabetic Index shown. Benign in category 216 indicates all of the diagnosis codes in this category are benign (Schraffenberger 2010, 79, 84).

103. a   Category 996 includes codes that identify complication in the use of artivicial substitutes or natural sources. To classify a mechanical reason for revision of a joint replacement, ICD-9-CM diagnosis codes 996.40 through 996.49 are available. In addition to one of these codes, the patient should also be assigned a code from V43.60 through V43.69 to identify the joint previously replaced by prosthesis. A directional note under the subcategory directs the coder to the additional V code (Schraffenberger 2010, 293–294).

104. b   Code 434.91 is assigned when the diagnosis states stroke or cerebrovascular accident (CVA) without further specification. Conditions resulting from a CVA, such as aphasia or hemiplegia, should be coded only if stated to be residual or present at the time of discharge. Do not code if these conditions are transient and resolved by the time of discharge (Schraffenberger 2010, 157–158).

105. a   Intravascular ultrasound is the correct answer. Per CPT guidelines, code 33880, angiography of the thoracic aorta, fluoroscopic guidance in delivery of the endovascular components, and preprocedure diagnostic imaging are all included in the repair code. Intravascular ultrasound may be reported separately if performed (AHIMA 2010a, 584).

106. a Acute respiratory failure, code 518.81, may be assigned as a principal or secondary diagnosis depending on the circumstances of the inpatient admission. Chapter-specific coding guidelines provide specific sequencing direction and take precedence over respiratory failure. Respiratory failure may be listed as a secondary diagnosis in that case. If respiratory failure occurs after admission, it would be listed as a secondary diagnosis (Schraffenberger 2010, 175).

107. d Adverse effects can occur in situation in which medication is administered properly and prescribed correctly in both therapeutic and diagnostic procedures. An adverse effect can occur when everything is done correctly. The first listed diagnosis is the manifestation or the nature of the adverse effect, such as the hematuria. Locate the drug in the Substance column of the Table of Drugs and Chemicals in the Alphabetic Index to Diseases. Select the E code for the drug from the Therapeutic Use column of the Table of Drugs and Chemicals. Use of the E code is mandatory when coding adverse effects (Schraffenberger 2010, 285).

108. c Hospitals, physicians, insurers, and health services researchers may use the codes. See the Introduction to Category III codes (AMA 2010b, 519; AHIMA 2010a, 616).

109. c Use a fifth digit of "1" to designate the first episode of care (regardless of facility site) for a newly diagnosed myocardial infarction. The fifth digit "1" is assigned regardless of the number of times a patient may be transferred during the initial episode of care (Schraffenberger 2010, 147).

110. b (Johns 2007, chapter 7)

111. a All claims involving inpatient admissions to general acute care hospitals or other facilities that are subject to law or regulation mandating collection of present on admission information. *Present on admission* (POA) is defined as present at the time the order for inpatient admission occurs. Conditions that develop during an outpatient encounter, including emergency department, observation, or outpatient surgery, are considered POA. Any condition that occurs after admission is not consider a POA condition (Schraffenberger 2010, 601).

112. b (Johns 2007, chapter 7)

113. b *Septicemia* generally refers to a systemic disease associated with the presence of pathological microorganisms or toxins in the blood, which can include bacteria, viruses, fungi, or other organisms. Code 038.11 is assigned for septicemia with staphylococcus aureus. Because abdominal pain is a symptom of diverticulisis, only the diverticulitis of the colon (562.11) is coded (Schraffenberger 2010, 68–69; Hart et al. 2009, 193).

114. c When the primary malignant neoplasm previously removed by surgery or eradicated by radiotherapy or chemotheraphy recurs, the primary malignant code for the site is assigned, unless the Alphabetic Index directs otherwise (Schraffenberger 2010, 90).

115. a The ventral hernia is coded as the primary or first listed diagnosis. The repair of the hernia is not coded because it was not performed; however, code 54.11 is assigned to describe the extent of the procedure, which is an exploratory laparotomy. The V64.3 is coded to indicate the cancelled procedure. Code 427.89 is also coded to describe the bradycardia that the patient develops during the procedure (Schraffenberger 2010, 40–41).

116. b *V codes* are diagnosis codes and indicate a reason for healthcare encounter (Schraffenberger 2010, 321).

117. b The fracture is the principle diagnosis, with the contusions as a secondary diagnosis. The fracture is what required the most treatment. Procedures for the reduction, débridement, and external fixation device would all need to be coded (Schraffenberger 2010, 265–266).

118. d Begin with the main term Revision; pacemaker site; chest (Kuehn 2010, 26).

119. a Code 54401 is correct because the prosthesis is self-contained (Kuehn 2010, 26).

120. d Modifier –24 is used for unrelated evaluation and management service by the same physician during a postoperative period (Kuehn 2010, 53).

121. d If the patient is admitted in withdrawal or if withdrawal develops after admission, the withdrawal code is designated as the principle diagnosis. The code for substance abuse/dependence is listed second (Schraffenberger 2010, 120).

122. a The anemia would be sequenced first based on principle diagnosis guidelines (Schraffenberger 2010, 48).

123. d The patient was admitted for the senile cataract and the procedures were completed for that condition. This follows the UHDDS guidelines for principle diagnosis selection. There is also no causal relationship given between the diabetes and the cataract, so 250.50 would be incorrect (Schraffenberger 2010, 100–101, 132).

124. d Patient was admitted for COPD, so this is listed as the principle diagnosis. Code 491.21 is used when the medical record includes documentation of COPD with acute exacerbation. ICD-9-CM presumes a cause-and-effect relationship and classifies chronic kidney disease with hypertension as hypertensive chronic kidney disease, assign code 403.91, however the code also at category 403 directs the coder to also code the chronic renal failure 585.9 (Schraffenberger 2010, 142–143, 174).

125. c The closed reduction of the fracture is coded first following principle procedure guidelines. The laceration repair is also coded. When more than one classification of wound repair is performed, all codes are reported, with the code for the most complicated procedure listed first (Kuehn 2010, 29, 105).

126. c A bronchoscopy with brushings and washings is considered a diagnostic bronchoscopy and not a biopsy. Code 31623 specifies brushings and 31622 is selected for washings (Kuehn 2010, 129).

127. d Modifiers are appended to the code to provide more information or to alert the payer that a payment change is required. Modifier –55 is used to identify the physician provided only postoperative care services for a particular procedure (Kuehn 2010, 270, 273).

128. b Begin at main term: Destruction, hemorrhoid, thermal. Thermal includes infrared coagulation (Kuehn 2010, 26, 156).

129. b A *logic-based encoder* prompts the user through a variety of questions and choices based on the clinical terminology entered. The coder selects the most accurate code for a service or condition (and any possible complications or comorbidities) (LaTour and Eichenwald Maki 2010, 400).

130. a Main term: Depression, subterm: recurrent with fifth digit of "3" for severe, without mention of psychotic behavior (Schraffenberger 2010, 115).

131. c Main term for procedure: Esophagoscopy, subterm: with closed biopsy (Schraffenberger 2010, 38–39).

132. d Codes for symptoms, signs, and ill-defined conditions are not to be used as the principle diagnosis when a related definitive diagnosis has been established. The flank pain would not be coded because it is a symptom of the calculus (Schraffenberger 2010, 51).

133. c Main term for diagnosis: Incontinence, subterm: stress. Main term for procedure: Suspension, subterm: urethra (Schraffenberger 2010, 10–11).

134. c Index the main term of hernia repair; inguinal; incarcerated. The age of the patient and the fact that the hernia is not recurrent make the choice 49507 (Kuehn 2010, 26, 156–158).

135. c Begin with the main term of Hernia repair; incisional. The fact that the hernia is recurrent, done via a laparoscope and is reducible make the choice 49656. Notice that the use of mesh is included in the code (Kuehn 2010, 26, 156–158).

136. b Main term of Hysteroscopy; lysis; adhesions (Kuehn 2010, 26, 174).

137. d In the abdomen, peritoneum, and omentum subsection, the exploratory laparotomy is a separate procedure and should not be reported when it is part of a larger procedure. The code of 49000 is not reported because laparotomy is the approach to the surgery. The code 58720 includes bilateral so the modifier –50 is not necessary to report (Kuehn 2010, 149).

138. c Dialysis, end-stage renal disease. Code 90966 is for end-stage renal disease (ESRD) related services for home dialysis per full month, for patients 20 years of age and older (Smith 2010, 203).

139. a Electrocardiography, evaluation. Code 93005 is the technical or facility code for reporting the tracing only, without interpretation and report. Code 93000 is a global code which includes the tracing and interpretation and report. Code 93010 includes the professional component by a physician with the interpretation and report. It is inappropriate to bill 93000 with 93010 and would be considered unbundling (Smith 2010, 206–208).

140. c Code 97113, Therapeutic procedure, 1 or more areas, each 15 minutes aquatic therapy with therapeutic exercises, is billable per 15 minutes of therapy. The patient was treated for 30 minutes, therefore, code 97113 should be reported twice. Modifier –50 is not applicable since the service is not a bilateral procedure (Smith 2010, 214).

Domain 4

141. a (Johns 2007, chapter 7)

142. b (Garvin 2010, 62, 203)

143. c (Johns 2007, chapter 7)

144. a (Johns 2007, chapter 7)

145. c (Johns 2007, chapter 7)

146. d (Johns 2007, chapter 7)

147. b (Johns 2007, chapter 7)

148. a (Johns 2007, chapter 7)

149. a (Johns 2007, chapter 7)

150. b (Johns 2007, chapter 7)

151. c (Johns 2007, chapter 7)

152. b (Johns 2007, chapter 7)

153. c (HHS 2003)

154. a (Johns 2007, chapter 7)

155. a (Russo 2010, chapter 3)

156. c (Garvin 2010, 62, 203)

157. c (Johns 2007, chapter 7)

158. a (Johns 2007, chapter 7)

159. d (Johns 2007, chapter 7)

160. d (Johns 2007, chapter 7)

Domain 5

161. b (Johns 2007, chapter 4)

162. b (Johns 2007, chapter 19)

163. c (Johns 2007, chapter 6)

164. d (Johns 2007, chapter 4)

165. c (Johns 2007, chapter 4)

166. b (Johns 2007, chapter 4)

167. c (Johns 2007, chapter 8)

168. d (Johns 2007, chapter 4)

169. a (Johns 2007, chapter 2)

170. c (Johns 2007, chapter 4)

171. c (Johns 2007, chapter 4)

172. c (Johns 2007, chapter 5)

Domain 6

173. b *Confidentiality* is a legal ethical concept that establishes the healthcare provider's responsibility for protecting health records and other personal and private information from unauthorized use or disclosure (Brodnik et al. 2009, 6).

174. d The UHCDA suggests that decision-making priority for an individual's next-of-kin be as follows: Spouse, adult child, parent, adult sibling, or if no one is available who is so related to the individual, authority may be granted to "an adult who exhibited special care and concern for the individual" (Brodnik et al. 2009, 113).

175. b A subpoena is a direct command that requires an individual or a representative of an organization to appear in court or to present an object to the court (Odom-Wesley et al. 2009, 57).

176. a Employees in departments such as the business office, information systems, HIM, and infection control, who are not involved directly in patient care, will vary in their need to access patient information. The HIPAA "minimum necessary" principle must be applied to determine what access employees should legitimately have to PHI (45 CFR 164.502 (b); Brodnik et al. 2009, 245).

177. a The law permits a presumption of consent during emergency situations, regardless of whether the patient is an adult or minor (Brodnik et al. 2009, 99).

178. b In order to practice medicine, a physician must graduate from an approved medical school and pass a state-based licensure exam. This exam allows a physician to obtain a drug enforcement administration number, which is required to prescribe medications and practice medicine (Brodnik et al. 2009, 348).

179. b State laws have developed requirements for certain deaths, such as accidental, homicidal, suicidal, sudden, and suspicious in nature to be reported, usually to the medical examiner or coroner. In addition, deaths as a result of abortion or induced termination of pregnancy are also reportable (Brodnik et al. 2009, 279).

180. b The physician would not have access to records of patient he or she is not treating unless the physician is performing designated healthcare operations such as research, peer review, or quality management. Otherwise the physician would need to have an authorization from the patient (Brodnik et al. 2009, 245).

181. b (Johns 2007, chapter 15)

182. a (Servais 2008, 1)

183. b (Johns 2007, chapter 14)

184. a *Nonmaleficence* means not harming others (Johns 2007, chapter 14).

185. b (Johns 2007, chapter 2)

186. b (Johns 2007, chapter 3)

187. c (Johns 2007, chapter 3)

188. b Individuals should be informed how covered entities use or disclose PHI (Johns 2007, chapter 4).

189. a (Johns 2007, chapter 5)

190. c (Johns 2007, chapter 3)

191. b (Johns 2007, chapter 13)

192. b (Johns 2007, chapter 15)

193. b During discovery both parties use various strategies to discover information about a case. The primary focus is to determine the strength of the opposing party's case (Johns 2007, chapter 15).

194. c (Johns 2007, chapter 15)

195. a (Johns 2007, chapter 15)

196. c *Subpoena duces tecum* is a written document directing individuals or organizations to furnish relevant documents and records (Johns 2007, chapter 15; AHIMA 2010b, 283).

197. c (Johns 2007, chapter 15)

198. a (Johns 2007, chapter 15)

199. b (Johns 2007, chapter 15)

200. b (Johns 2007, chapter 15)

Certified Coding Associate
Exam Preparation

Answer Key
Practice Exam 1

Domain 1

1. c (Odom-Wesley et al. 2009, 310)

2. c *Vocabulary standards* establish common definitions for medical terms to encourage consistent descriptions of an individual's condition in the health record (Johns 2007, chapter 5).

3. a The consultation report documents the clinical opinion of a physician other than the primary or attending physician. The report is based on the consulting physician's examination of the patient and a review of his or her health record (Johns 2007, chapter 3).

4. a (Johns 2007, chapter 3)

5. a The *discharge summary* is a concise account of the patient's illness, course of treatment, response to treatment, and condition at the time the patient is discharged (Johns 2007, chapter 2).

6. c The nature and duration of the symptoms that caused the patient to seek medical attention as stated in the patient's own words (Odom-Wesley et al. 2009, 331).

7. a *Clinical information* is data that is related to the patient's diagnosis or treatment in a healthcare facility (Odom-Wesley et al. 2009, 55).

8. d Financial data includes details about the patient's occupation, employer, and insurance coverage (Odom-Wesley et al. 2009, 42).

9. c The *Subjective, Objective, Assessment, Plan (SOAP) notes* are part of the problem-oriented medical records (POMR) approach most commonly used by physicians and other healthcare professionals. SOAP notes are intended to improve the quality and continuity of client services by enhancing communication among healthcare professionals (Odom-Wesley et al. 2009, 217).

10. b The Uniform Ambulatory Care Data Set (UACDS) includes data elements specific to ambulatory care, such as the reason for the encounter with the healthcare provider (LaTour and Eichenwald Maki 2010, 166).

11. a The transfer or referral form provides document communication between caregivers in multiple healthcare settings. It is important that a patient's treatment plan be consistent as the patient moves through the healthcare delivery system (Odom-Wesley et al. 2009, 131).

12. b Synthroid is given to patients to augment or replace small levels of thyroid hormone, thyroxine.

13. c *Klebsiella* is a type of gram-negative bacteria that can cause infections, including

pneumonia, in healthcare settings (HHS 2010).

14. c The total size of a removed lesion, including margins, is needed for accurate coding. This information is best provided in the operative report. The pathology report typically provides the specimen size rather than the size of the excised lesion. Because the specimen tends to shrink, this is not an accurate measurement (Kuehn 2010, 108).

15. b Protonix is used to treat patients with erosive esophagitis associated with GERD. It decreases the accumulation of acid in the stomach (drugs.com, 2009).

16. d Status asthmaticus is an acute asthmatic attack in which the degree of bronchial obstruction is not relieved by usual treatments such as epinephrine or aminophylline. A patient in status asthmaticus fails to respond to therapy. Only a physician can diagnose status asthmaticus. If a coder suspects the condition based on the symptoms documented in the record, the coder should query the physician about the documentation for status asthmaticus (CMS 2010c, Section I, C, 8).

17. a *Hypokalemia* is defined as abnormally low potassium concentration in the blood (Dorland's, 895).

18. b A complete medical history documents the patient's current complaints and symptoms and lists the patient's past medical, social, and family history (Johns 2007, chapter 2).

19. b The ICD-9-CM *Official Guidelines for Coding and Reporting* indicate that when a physician qualifies a diagnostic statement as "rule out," the condition qualified in that statement should not be coded as if it existed. Rather, the condition should be coded to the highest level of certainty, such as the signs and symptoms the patient exhibits (CMS 2010c, Section IV).

20. a *Medical necessity* is defined as accepted healthcare services and supplies provided by healthcare providers, appropriate to the evaluation and treatment of a disease, condition, illness, or injury and consistent with the applicable standard of care (AHIMA 2010b).

Domain 2

21. b The benefit of concurrent review is that content or authentication issues can be identified at the time of patient care and rectified in a timely manner (Johns 2007, 776).

22. c The HIM manager may compare organizational data with external data from peer groups to determine best practices (Johns 2007, chapter 11).

23. d Surveyors review the documentation of patient care services to determine whether the standards for care are being met (Johns 2007, chapter 2).

24. c Participating organizations must follow the Medicare Conditions of Participation to receive federal funds from the Medicare program for services rendered (Johns 2007, 86).

25. c Compliance with state licensing laws is required in order for healthcare organizations to remain in operation (Johns 2007, chapter 3).

26. b The pathology report describes specimens examined by the pathologist (Johns 2007, chapter 2).

27. b (Johns 2007, chapter 8)

28. a According to the Joint Commission, the physical exam must be completed within 24 hours of admission (Odom-Wesley et al. 2009, 353).

29. c According to the Joint Commission, except in emergency situations, every surgical patient's chart must include a report of a complete history and physical conducted no more than seven days before the surgery is to be performed (Odom-Wesley et al. 2009, 150).

30. d Quality improvement (QI) programs have been in place in hospitals for years and have been required by the Medicare/Medicaid programs and accreditation standards. QI programs have covered medical staff as well as nursing and other departments or processes (LaTour and Eichenwald Maki 2010, 33).

31. c As part of the decision making process, the HIM director should analyze the problem and develop alternative solutions (Johns 2007, chapter 20).

32. a The coder is not following established policies (Johns 2007, chapter 6).

33. a (LaTour and Eichenwald Maki 2010, 182)

34. c Progress notes are chronological statements about the patient's response to treatment during his or her stay at the facility (Kuehn 2010, 10).

Domain 3

35. d Index fracture, femur, epiphysis, capital. Fifth digits are required for further classification of a specific condition. Many publishers include special symbols and/or color highlighting to identify codes that require a fourth or fifth digit (Schraffenberger 2010, 7).

36. d Index eruption, teeth/tooth, neonatal. Some main terms are followed by a list of indented subterms (modifiers) that affect the selection of an appropriate code for a given diagnosis. The subterms form individual line entries arranged in alphabetical order and printed in a regular type beginning with a lowercase letter. Subterms are indented on standard indention to the right under the main term. More specific subterms are further indented after the preceding subterm (Schraffenberger 2010, 12).

37. a CPT code 21012 describes excision of a subcutaneous soft tissue tumor of the face or scalp, greater than 2 cm. and is appropriately coded when the tumor is removed from the subcutaneous tissue rather than subgaleal or intramuscular. Simple and intermediate closure of the wound is included in the procedure for the excision in the musculoskeletal section of CPT (AMA 2010a, 28–29; AMA 2010b, 86, 92).

38. c Fine needle aspiration with image guidance is coded with 10022. Instructional note directs coder to assign 19295 for placement of localization clip during a breast biopsy. Add radiology code 76942 for supervision and interpretation of ultrasound guidance for localization clip guidance. See instructional notes following code 10022 (AMA 2010a, 21, 25).

39. a Index Disease, Lou Gehrig's or Lou Gehrig's disease. Amyotropic lateral sclerosis is another name for Lou Gehrig's disease. Many diseases carry the name of a person, or an eponym. The main terms for eponyms are located in the Alphabetic Index under the eponym or the disease, syndrome, or disorder (Schraffenberger 2010, 13).

40. d ICD-9-CM classifies cardiac pacemakers to code 37.8: Insertion, replacement, removal, and revision of pacemaker device. In coding initial insertion of a permanent pacemaker, two codes are required—one for the pacemaker (37.80–37.83) and one for the lead (37.70–37.74) (Schraffenberger 2010, 165).

41. a When a pacemaker is replaced with another pacemaker, only the replaced pacemaker is coded (37.85–37.87). Removal of the old pacemaker is not coded (Schraffenberger 2010, 165).

42. b Index block, left, with right bundle branch block. Right and left bundle branch block is inclusive of one code. It is inappropriate to assign a code for right (426.4) and left (426.3) bundle branch block when a combination code includes both the right and left (Schraffenberger 2010, 167).

43. a Index fitting (of) pacemaker (cardiac). No procedure code exists in ICD-9-CM to describe reprogramming (Schraffenberger 2010, 165).

44. d SSS is the imprecise diagnosis with various characteristics treated with the insertion of a permanent cardiac pacemaker. The other three conditions are treated with cardioversion and different pharmacological therapy (Schraffenberger 2010, 154).

45. c Index bypass, internal mammary-coronary artery (single), double vessel (36.16). Internal mammary-coronary artery bypass is accomplished by loosening the internal mammary artery from its normal position and using the internal mammary artery to bring blood from the subclavian artery to the occluded coronary artery. Codes are selected based on whether one or both internal mammary arteries are used, regardless of the number of coronary arteries involved (Schraffenberger 2010, 164).

46. c The Judkins technique provides x-ray imaging of the coronary arteries by introducing one catheter into the femoral artery with maneuvering up into the left coronary artery orifice, followed by a second catheter guided up into the right coronary artery, and subsequent injection of a contrast material (Schraffenberger 2010, 166).

47. a V58.83, Encounter for therapeutic drug monitoring, is the correct code to use when a patient visit if for the sole purpose of undergoing a laboratory test to measure the drug level in the patient's blood or urine or to measure a specific function to assess the effectiveness of the drug. V58.83 may be used alone if the monitoring is for a drug that the patient is on for only a brief period, not long term. However, there is a Use Additional Code note after code V58.83 to remind the coder to use the additional code for any associated long-term drug use with codes V58.61–V58.69 (Schraffenberger 2010, 338).

48. c Code 43761 is assigned to report repositioning of a naso- or oro-gastric feeding tube through the duodenum. An instructional note guides the coder to report code 76000 when image guidance is performed (AMA 2010a, 112; AMA 2010b, 222).

49. d Code 49450 includes replacement of gastrostomy or cecostomy tube, percutaneous, under fluoroscopic guidance including contrast injections(s), image documentation and report. Therefore, it would not be appropriate to add code 76000 for fluoroscopic guidance, which is already included in the procedure code (AMA 2010a, 122).

50. c Index Ovum, blighted

51. b Index Abortion, threatened 640.0. Refer to the ICD-9-CM Tabular (640–649) for the correct fifth digit of "3", antepartum condition, not delivered.

52. a Index Delivery, Cesarean, poor dilation, cervix 661.0. Refer to the ICD-9-CM Tabular (660–669) for the correct fifth digit of "1", delivered, with or without mention of antepartum condition. Outcome of delivery, single, liveborn. Cesarean section, low uterine segment.

53. b Index Rash, diaper. ICD-9-CM classifies dermatitis to categories 690–694. Atopic dermatitis and related conditions are specific to category 691. Fourth-digit subcategories include diaper or napkin rash and other atopic dermatitis and related conditions (Schraffenberger 2010, 226).

54. a Index Ingrowing, nail (finger) (toe) (infected)

55. b Index Lymphadenitis, acute

56. b Index Osteoarthrosis, localized, primary. For category 715, refer to the table for the fifth digit of "5" for pelvic region and thigh.

57. a Index Chondromalacia, patella

58. d Index Paget's disease, bone. The main terms for eponyms are located in the Alphabetic Index under the eponym or the disease, syndrome, or disorder (Schraffenberger 2010, 13).

59. d Index Osteomyelitis, acute or subacute. Refer to the table in the index for the fifth digit "5", ankle and foot. Infection, staphylococcal NEC.

60. b Index Anemia, aplastic, due to, antineoplastic chemotherapy. A coder should always assign the most specific type of anemia. Anemia due to chemotherapy is often aplastic (AHA 2009a, 20).

61. c Index Exam, well baby. Premature, infant NEC. Refer to table in Tabular for fifth digit of "0" to note unspecified birth weight (AHA 2009c, 15).

62. d Index Dysfunction, diastolic (AHA 2009d, 7).

63. d Index Embolization, artery, by, endovascular approach. Angiography, intra-abdominal NEC (AHA 2009e, 7).

64. c Index Transplant, stem cell, allogeneic (hematopoietic) (AHA 2009d, 9).

65. c Use this code when the diagnosis is specified as a certain type of "benign mammary dysplasia" and in this case, "ductal" hyperplasia. Index Hyperplasia, breast, ductal, atypical.

66. c Index Bunionectomy or Mayo operation, bunionectomy. The main terms for eponyms are located in the Alphabetic Index under the eponym or the disease, syndrome, operation, or disorder (Schraffenberger 2010, 13).

67. b Index Lobectomy, lung, segmental (with resection of adjacent lobes), thoracoscopic. Segmental includes the complete excision of a lobe of the lung.

68. d Index Cholecystectomy (total), laparoscopic

69. c Index Cystoscopy (transurethral), with biopsy

70. d Index Insertion, tissue expander (skin) NEC, breast

Domain 4

71. b An *encoder* is a computer software program designed to assist coders in assigning appropriate clinical codes. An encoder helps ensure accurate reporting of diagnoses and procedures (LaTour and Eichenwald Maki 2010, 318–319).

72. b The RBRVS system is the federal government's payment system for physicians. It is a system of classifying health services based on the cost of furnishing physicians' services in different settings, the skill and training levels required to perform the services, and the time and risk involved (Casto and Layman 2009, 157; Brown 2009).

73. c *Unbundling* is the practice of coding services separately that should be coded together as a package because all parts are included within one code and therefore, one price. Unbundling done deliberately could be considered fraud (Kuehn 2010, 335).

74. b *CPT Assistant* is considered the official source for CPT coding guidance on how to assign a CPT code. The American Medical Association publishes the guidance monthly (AMA 2010b).

75. b Unbundling occurs when a panel code exists and the individual tests are reported rather than the panel code (AMA 2010b, 389).

76. a Reporting additional test codes that overlap codes in a panel allows the coder to assign all appropriate codes for services provided. It is inappropriate to assign additional panel codes when all codes in the panel are not performed. Reporting individual lab codes is appropriate when all codes in a panel have not been provided (AMA 2010b, 389).

77. a The coder should assign the most comprehensive code to describe the entire procedure performed. When a code describes the entire service provided the coder should not code each component separately. Assigning additional codes inherent to the main code would be a form of unbundling (Hazelwood and Venable 2010, 300).

78. b CMS developed the NCCI to control improper coding practices leading to inappropriate payments in Part B claims (CMS 2010a).

79. c AHA's *Coding Clinic* for ICD-9-CM is a quarterly publication of the Central Office on ICD-9-CM, which allows coders to submit a request for coding advice through the coding publication.

80. b CMS developed MUEs to prevent providers from billing units in excess and receiving inappropriate payments. This new editing was the result of the outpatient prospective payment system which pays providers passed on the HCPCS/CPT code and units. Payment is directly related to units for specified HCPCS/CPT codes assigned to an ambulatory payment classification (CMS 2010b).

Domain 5

81. b (Johns 2007, chapter 8)

82. a (Johns 2007, chapter 9)

83. a Role-based access control (RBAC) is a control system in which access decisions are based on the roles of individual users as part of an organization (Brodnik et al. 2009, 211).

84. c As important as firewalls are to the overall security of health information systems, they cannot protect a system from all types of attacks. Many viruses, for example, can hide within documents that will not be stopped by a firewall (Brodnik et al. 2009, 218).

85. d EDI allows the transfer (incoming and outgoing) of information directly from one computer to another by using flexible, standard formats (Johns 2007, chapter 4).

86. c A software interface is a computer program that allows different applications to communicate and exchange data (Johns 2007, chapter 4).

Domain 6

87. c The designated record set includes health records that are used to make decisions about the individual (Johns 2007, chapter 7).

88. a The covered entity must provide access to the personal health information in the form or format requested when it is readily producible in such form for format. When it is not readily producible in the form or format requested, it must be produced in a readable hard-copy form or such other form or format agreed to by the covered entity and the individual (Johns 2007, chapter 7).

89. c (Johns 2007, chapter 2)

90. c (Johns 2007, chapter 8)

91. b (Johns 2007, chapter 15)

92. a (Servais 2008, chapter 5)

93. b (Johns 2007, chapter 19)

94. d Health records in all formats are covered by HIPAA (Johns 2007, chapter 15).

95. d Privileged communication is a legal concept designed to protect the confidentiality between two parties (Brodnik et al. 2009, 6).

96. c Generally, if the patient is a minor at the time of treatment or hospitalization but has reached the age of majority at the time the authorization for access or disclosure of information is signed, the patient's authorization is legally required (Brodnik et al. 2009, 243).

97. c English common law is the primary source of many legal rules and principles and was based initially on tradition and custom. Common law, also known as judge-made law or case law, is regularly referred to as unwritten law originating from court decisions where no applicable statute exists (LaTour and Eichenwald Maki 2010, 272).

98. d HIM professionals must factor several criteria into their decision making. Ethicists provide assistance in this process. When faced with an ethical issue, the HIM professional should evaluate the ethical problem following these steps: Determine the facts; consider the values and obligations of others; consider the choices that are both justified and not justified; and identify prevention options. When a decision must be made about an issue and not identified following the steps, the decision most likely will be based on an individual's narrow moral perspective of right or wrong (LaTour and Eichenwald Maki 2010, 318).

99. c When a state law is more stringent than a federal law, hospitals must comply with both (Odom-Wesley et al. 2009, 68).

100. c A facility may maintain a facility directory of patients being treated. HIPAA's Privacy Rule permits the facility to maintain in its directory the following information about an individual if the individual has not objected: name, location in the facility, and condition described in general terms. This information may be disclosed to persons who ask for the individual by name (Brodnik et al. 2009, 171).

Certified Coding Associate
Exam Preparation

Answer Key
Practice Exam 2

Domain 1

1. b (Johns 2007, chapter 2)

2. a *Present on admission* is defined as present at the time the order for inpatient admission occurs (CMS 2010c, Appendix I).

3. b Medical history documents the patient's current complaints and symptoms and lists the patient's past medical, personal, and family history. The physical examination report represents the attending physician's assessment of the patient's current health status (Johns 2007, chapter 3).

4. b (Odom-Wesley et al. 2009, 150)

5. a (Johns 2007, 62)

6. d The physical examination report represents the attending physician's assessment of the patient's current health status (Johns 2007, 54).

7. c A pathology report usually includes descriptions of the tissue from a gross or macroscopic level and representative cells at the microscopic level along with interpretive findings (Johns 2007, 66).

8. b A *pathology report* is a document that contains the diagnosis determined by examining cells and tissues under a microscope. The report may also contain information about the size, shape, and appearance of a specimen as it looks to the naked eye (Odom-Wesley et al. 2009, 171).

9. a In 1997, the Joint Commission introduced the ORYX initiative to integrate outcomes data and other performance measurement data into its accreditation processes (LaTour and Eichenwald Maki 2010, 170).

10. a *Abstracting* is the function of compiling the pertinent information from the medical record based on predetermined data sets (LaTour and Eichenwald Maki 2010, 91).

11. b One of the five categories of health informatics standards is vocabulary standards which purpose is to establish uniform definitions for clinical terms (Odom-Wesley et al. 2009, 310).

12. b Code description for 659.5 in ICD-9-CM includes the first pregnancy in a woman who will be 35 or older at the expected date of delivery.

13. a (Hazelwood and Venable 2010, 221)

14. c (Hazelwood and Venable 2010, 209)

15. b (Hazelwood and Venable 2010, 73)

16. b Retrovir is an antiretroviral which is used to treat viral infections, including HIV infections, which causes AIDS (drugs.com, 2010a).

17. d (Hazelwood and Venable 2010, 169)

18. a *Histology* refers to the tissue type of a lesion. The histology of tissue is determined by a pathologist and documented in the pathology report (Johns 2007, 58).

19. c Haldol is used to treat symptoms of schizophrenia (drugs.com, 2010b).

Domain 2

20. c The American College of Surgeons started its Hospital Standardization Program in 1918 (Johns 2007, 482).

21. c All entries must be legible and complete, and must be authenticated and dated promptly by the person (identified by name and discipline) who is responsible for ordering, providing, or evaluating the service furnished (42 CFR 482.24).

22. d (Johns 2007, 91–92)

23. c (Russo 2010, chapter 6)

24. c (AHIMA 2008b, 83–88)

25. b (AHIMA 2005)

26. d (Gelzer et al. 2008, 11)

27. a The physician principally responsible for the patient's hospital care writes and signs the discharge summary (Odom-Wesley et al. 2009, 200).

28. a *Autoauthentication* is a policy that allows the physician or provider to state in advance that dictated and transcribed reports should automatically be considered approved and signed when the physician does not make corrections within a certain period of time. Another variation of autoauthentication is that physicians authorize the HIM department to send a weekly list of documents needing signatures. The list is then signed and returned to the HIM department (LaTour and Eichenwald Maki 2010, 213).

29. d The discharge summary must be completed within 30 days after discharge for most patients but within 24 hours for patients transferred to other facilities. Discharge summaries are not always required for patients who are hospitalized for less than 48 hours (Odom-Wesley et al. 2009, 200).

30. a The Joint Commission, Commission on Accreditation of Rehabilitation Facilities, and

the National Committee for Quality Assurance are all acceptable accrediting bodies for behavioral healthcare settings (Odom-Wesley et al. 2009, 447).

31. b The purpose of *identifier standards* are to establish methods for assigning unique identifier to individual patients, healthcare professionals, healthcare provider organizations, and healthcare vendors and suppliers (Odom-Wesley et al. 2009, 311).

32. c State licensure agencies have regulations that are modeled after the Medicare Conditions of Participation and Joint Commission standards. States conduct annual surveys to determine the hospital's continued compliance with licensure standards (Odom-Wesley et al. 2009, 287).

33. d Medicare-certified home healthcare also uses a standardized patient assessment instrument called the OASIS (Johns 2007, 77).

Domain 3

34. c The residual condition or nature of the late effect is sequenced first, followed by the cause of the late effect (Hazelwood and Venable 2010, 55).

35. c The residual condition or nature of the late effect is sequenced first, followed by the cause of the late effect. Late effect exceptions occur when the late effect code has been expanded at the fourth- and fifth-digit level to include the manifestations. In this case, only one code is necessary to describe both the residual condition and cause of the late effect (Hazelwood and Venable 2010, 56).

36. a Conditions that are integral to the disease process should not be assigned as additional codes. The nausea and vomiting are integral to the disease, gastroenteritis (Hazelwood and Venable 2010, 60).

37. d Review Tabular Index: Findings, abnormal, without diagnosis, prostate specific antigen (PSA), 790.93, or Elevation, prostate specific antigen (PSA), 790.93 (Hazelwood and Venable 2010, 61).

38. b Near-syncope and nausea are both signs and symptoms and therefore not integral to the other. Both conditions should be coded (Hazelwood and Venable 2010, 63).

39. d The index may mislead the coder to a nonspecific code. In this example, when the coder references "Abnormal" and subheading "glucose", the coder is directed to code 790.29. The coder should always reference the Tabular to verify the code. During verification, the coder will see the selection for code 790.22, which accurately describes the specific abnormal finding of glucose tolerance test (Hazelwood and Venable 2010, 66).

40. c Pneumonia, unspecified is assigned 486 in the index. Cough is integral to pneumonia and should not be coded separately (Hazelwood and Venable 2010, 66).

41. a   Code signs and symptoms when a condition is *ruled out*, which means the condition has been proven not to exist. The code for seizures (780.39) is assigned when a more specific diagnosis cannot be made even after all the facts bearing on the case have been investigated (Hazelwood and Venable 2010, 60–66).

42. c   Index Incontinence, stress, male NEC 788.32. Category 788.3x indicates incontinence of urine with the fifth digit specific to different types such as urge, stress, mixed, and others (Hazelwood and Venable 2010, 65–66).

43. d   Abdominal pain includes fifth digits to identify the specific parts of the abdomen affected. Nausea and vomiting is a category common to stomach upset. The fifth digits provide specificity. Nausea and vomiting are coded together with a combination code when both exist. Diarrhea usually is a symptom of some other disorder or of a more severe disease, in which case it should not be coded separately. It is often accompanied by vomiting and various other symptoms that should be coded when present. Because a distinct disease is not available in this case, all the symptoms should be coded (Hazelwood and Venable 2010, 64–66).

44. a   Bronchiectasis (fusiform) (postinfectious) (recurrent) is an example of a diagnosis statement with nonessential modifiers noted with parentheses marks. The parentheses may or may not be present in a statement for the diagnosis or procedure in ICD-9-CM coding (Schraffenberger 2010, 27).

45. c   Per individual payer guidelines, review should be done of the post-op period because the diagnostic procedure was done. If the criteria are met, modifier –58 might be appropriate. The lesions were not described as primary neoplasm; therefore, code 162.2 is not accurate. The CPT code 31623–59 for bronchial washings is incorrect because the lesions were identified by this means in a previous bronchoscopy, and this episode was for the laser treatment through a rigid scope (AHIMA 2010a, 695).

46. d   CPT code 33813 is the repair of the aortopulmonary septal defect, or window, which is a communication between the ascending aorta and the main pulmonary artery above the two distinct semilunar valves. A patent ductus arteriosus is a connection between the aorta and the pulmonary artery within the aortic arch, well above the heart. PDA closure is described by 33820–33824, based on the method used for closure. In this case, the physician divides the connection and suturing each of the defects closed. CPT 33824 describes this service for a 22-year-old patient (AHIMA, 2010a, 690).

47. b   Index Infarction, myocardium, anterolateral (wall) with fifth digit for initial episode (Schraffenberger 2010, 29).

48. d   Only confirmed cases of HIV infection/illness are reported whether inpatient or outpatient. 042, Human immunodeficiency virus [HIV] disease. Patients with HIV-related illness should be coded to category 042, which includes AIDS, AIDS-like syndrome, AIDS-related complex, and symptomatic HIV infection (Hazelwood and Venable 2010, 81).

49. b Connecting words or connecting terms are subterms that indicate a relationship between the main term and an associated condition or etiology in the Alphabetic Index. The connecting term "due to" connects the organism *E. coli* to the urinary tract infection. The instructional note "Use additional code" is found in the Tabular List of ICD-9-CM. This notation indicates that use of an additional code may provide a more complete picture of the diagnosis or procedure. The additional code should always be assigned if the health record provides supportive documentation. Infection, urinary (tract) Tabular List—use additional code to identify organism. Infection, *Escherichia coli* (Schraffenberger 2010, 23–24, 67).

50. b When a patient is admitted for the purpose of radiotherapy, chemotherapy, or immunotherapy and develops a complication, such as uncontrolled nausea and vomiting or dehydration, the principal diagnosis is the admission for radiotherapy (V58.0), the admission for the antineoplastic chemotherapy (V58.11), or the admission for the antineoplastic immunotherapy (V58.12). Additional codes would include the cancer and the complication(s) (Hazelwood and Venable 2010, 91).

51. c The terms *metastatic to* and *direct extension to* are used for classifying secondary malignant neoplasms in ICD-9-CM. For example, cancer described as "metastatic to a specific site" is interpreted as a secondary neoplasm of that site. The colon (153.9) is the primary site, and the lung (197.0) is the secondary site (Hazelwood and Venable 2010, 97).

52. a 038.11, Septicemia, staphylococcal aureus and 995.91, Sepsis. The "Code First" note following code 995.91 directs the coder to assign the code for the underlying infection first (Schraffenberger 2010, 68–69, 74).

53. c Diabetes (without complication) with fifth digit of "2" = type II, uncontrolled. 263.1 Malnutrition, mild not stated as related to diabetes (Schraffenberger 2010, 100–105).

54. d 288.00, Fever, neutropenic. Instructional note states to use additional code for any associated fever (780.61) (Schraffenberger 2010, 113).

55. b Because the patient has no other documented complaints, only the V code is appropriate (Hazelwood and Venable 2010, 47).

56. a CPT code 82270 describes a test for occult blood using feces source for the purpose of neoplasm screening with the use of three cards or single triple card for consecutive collection (AMA 2010b, 395).

57. b New technology is addressed by the Category III codes (AHIMA 2010a, 567).

58. c (AHIMA 2010a, 568; AMA 2010b)

59. b Because a separate procedure is considered a part of, and integral to, another, larger procedure, it is not coded when performed as part of the more extensive procedure. See Surgery Guidelines. It may, however, be coded when it is not performed as part of another, larger service, so answer "c" is not correct (AHIMA 2010a, 569).

60. b The AMA developed and maintains CPT. CMS developed and maintains HCPCS Level II codes (AHIMA 2010a, 569).

61. c Any physician may use the codes in any section of CPT (AHIMA 2010a, 570).

62. d See instructional notes preceding code 99217. In order to report these codes, the admission order must designate observation service. Whether or not the patient meets admission criteria or is admitted following surgery does not affect the observation code selection. If the patient is admitted and discharged on the same date, codes 99234–99236 are appropriate (AHIMA 2010a, 571).

63. b Documentation of history of use of drugs, alcohol, and/or tobacco is considered part of the social history. The review of systems is a part of the history of present illness. See E/M Services Guidelines, instructions for selecting a level of E/M service, in the CPT manual (AHIMA 2010a, 47).

64. c Tissue transplanted from one individual to another of the same species but different genotype is called an *allograft* or *allogeneic graft* (AHIMA 2010a, 575–576).

65. b See definitions preceding code 17311 in CPT *Professional Edition* (AMA 2010a, 77).

66. a The "with manipulation" code is used because the fracture was manipulated, even if the manipulation did not result in clinical anatomic alignment. See Musculoskeletal Guidelines, Definitions (AHIMA 2010a, 580).

67. d Index Incision and Drainage, shoulder, bursa, resulting in code 23031 (AHIMA 2010a, 580).

68. a If the tip of the catheter is manipulated, it is a selective catheterization. In the case of a nonselective catheterization, the tip of the catheter remains in either the aorta or the artery that was originally entered (AHIMA 2010a, 585).

69. c The only vessel coded is the final vessel entered. See instructional note preceding code 36000. Intermediate steps along the way are not reported (AHIMA 2010a, 585).

Domain 4

70. b Diagnosis codes are often the primary reason for a service to be considered covered or denied by the insurance company. Local and national policies include diagnosis codes that are used in software edits to automatically deny or approve processed claims. Denied services can be appealed and the record can be submitted to support medical necessity if the service fails the automated review (Schraffenberger 2010, 63).

71. b The NUBC was established with the goal of developing an acceptable, uniform bill that would consolidate the numerous billing forms hospitals were required to use (Schraffenberger 2010, 49, 60).

72. c The Uniform Hospital Discharge Data Set was promulgated by the US Department of Health, Education, and Welfare in 1974 as a minimum, common core of data on individual acute-care, short-term hospital discharges in Medicare and Medicaid programs. It sought to improve the uniformity and comparability of hospital discharge data. In 1985, the data was expanded to include all nonoutpatient settings (Schraffenberger 2010, 47–48, 60).

73. a For fiscal year 2008, Medicare adopted a severity-adjusted diagnosis-related groups system called Medicare Severity-DRGs (MS-DRGs). This was the most drastic revision to the DRG system in 24 years. The goal of the new MS-DRG system was to significantly improve Medicare's ability to recognize severity of illness in its inpatient hospital payments. The new system is projected to increase payments to hospitals for services provided to the sicker patients and decrease payments for treating less severely ill patients (Schraffenberger 2010, 56, 62).

74. a For any given patient in a MS-DRG, the hospital knows, in advance, the amount of reimbursement it will receive from Medicare. It is the responsibility of the hospital to ensure that its resource use is in line with the payment (Schraffenberger 2010, 56–57, 62).

75. d Medicare provides for additional payment for other factors related to a particular hospital's business. If the hospital treats a high percentage of low-income patients, it receives a percentage add-on payment applied to the MS-DRG adjusted base payment rate. This add-on payment, known as the disproportionate share hospital (DSH) adjustment, provides for a percentage increase in Medicare payments to hospitals that qualify under either of two statutory formulas designed to identify hospitals that serve these areas. Hospitals that have approved teaching hospitals also receive a percentage add-on payment for each Medicare discharged paid under IPPS, known as the indirect medical education (IME) adjustment. The percentage varies, depending on the ratio of residents to beds. Additional payments are made for new technologies or medical services that have been approved for special add-on payments. Finally, the costs incurred by a hospital for a Medicare beneficiary are evaluated to determine whether the hospital is eligible for an additional payment as an outlier case. This additional payment is designed to protect the hospital from large financial losses due to unusually expensive cases (Schraffenberger 2010, 57, 62).

76. b Congress directed HHS to conduct a three-year demonstration project using RACs to detect and correct improper payments in the Medicare traditional fee-for-service program. Congress further required HHS to make the RAC program permanent and nationwide by January 1, 2010 (Schraffenberger 2010, 59, 63).

77. d The UB-04 has space for six procedure codes and space for the associated date the procedure occurred (Schraffenberger 2010, 60, 468).

78. b Attending and consulting physicians have no bearing on the assignment of the MS-DRG and payment to the hospital (Schraffenberger 2010, 57).

79. b A total of 18 diagnosis codes may be reported on the UB-04 paper claim form locator 67 (Schraffenberger 2010, 50, 60).

Domain 5

80. b (HHS 2006a)

81. c Edit checks help ensure data integrity by allowing only reasonable and predetermined values to be entered into the computer (Johns 2007, chapter 19).

82. b When several people enter data in an EHR, you can define how users must enter data in specific fields to help maintain consistency. For example, an input mask for a form means that users can only enter the date in a specified format (MacDonald 2007, chapter 4).

83. c Automated systems for registering patients and tracking their encounters are commonly known as admission-discharge-transfer (ADT) systems (Johns 2007, chapter 17).

84. b (Johns 2007, chapter 16)

85. b *Computer-assisted coding* is defined as the use of computer software that automatically generates a set of medical codes for review, validation, and use based on the documentation from the various providers of healthcare (AHIMA 2010b, 62; LaTour and Eichenwald Maki 2010, 400).

Domain 6

86. b (LaTour and Eichenwald Maki 2010, 258)

87. a (AHIMA e-HIM Work Group on Medical Identity Theft 2008a, 63–69)

88. a (Johns 2007, chapter 14)

89. b *Beneficence* means promoting good (Johns 2007, chapter 14).

90. d (LaTour and Eichenwald Maki 2010, 284; 45 CFR 164.524)

91. b (Johns 2007, chapter 14)

92. d The distinction of psychotherapy notes is important due to HIPAA requirements that these notes may not be released unless specifically specified in an authorization (Odom-Wesley et al. 2009, 440).

93. d When a person or entity that willfully and knowingly violates the HIPAA Privacy Rule, a fine of not more than $250,000, not more than 10 years in jail, or both may be imposed (LaTour and Eichenwald Maki 2010, 292).

94. c No; the HIPAA Privacy Rule introduced the standard that individuals should be informed of how covered entities (CEs) use or disclose protected health information. This notice must be provided to an individual at his or her first contact with the CE (Brodnik et al. 2009, 165).

95. a (Brodnik et al. 2009, 167)

96. c The Privacy Rule's general requirement is that authorization must be obtained for uses and disclosure of protected health information created for research that includes treatment of the individual (Brodnik et al. 2009, 183).

97. a (Hazelwood and Venable 2010, 312; AHIMA 2008d)

98. b (Johns 2007, chapter 19)

99. c (NIST 2006, chapter 18)

100. c When a state law is more stringent than a federal law, hospitals must comply with both (Odom-Wesley et al. 2009, 68).

Certified Coding Associate
Exam Preparation

References and Resources

American Health Information Management Association. 2010a. *Clinical Coding Workout: Practice Exercises for Skill Development, 2010 Edition with Answers.* Chicago. AHIMA

American Health Information Management Association. 2010b. *Pocket Glossary of Health Information Management and Technology.* 2nd ed. Chicago: AHIMA.

American Health Information Management Association e-HIM Work Group on Medical Identity Theft. 2008a. Practice Brief: Mitigating medical identity theft. *Journal of AHIMA* 79(7).

American Health Information Management Association. 2008b. Practice brief: Managing an effective query process. *Journal of AHIMA* 79(10).

American Health Information Management Association. 2008c (Dec. 16). Communities of Practice: Medical Record Information.

American Health Information Management Association. 2008d (September). AHIMA's Code of Ethics.   http://www.ahima.org/about/ethics.asp.*

American Health Information Management Association. 2005. e-HIM Work Group on Maintaining the Legal EHR. "Update: Maintaining a Legally Sound Health Record—Paper and Electronic." *Journal of AHIMA* 76(10): 64A–L.

American Hospital Association. *Coding Clinic for ICD-9-CM* 2009a, 1Q:20. Chicago.

American Hospital Association. *Coding Clinic for ICD-9-CM* 2009b, 2Q:19. Chicago.

American Hospital Association. *Coding Clinic for ICD-9-CM* 2009c, 1Q:15. Chicago.

American Hospital Association. *Coding Clinic for ICD-9-CM* 2009d, 1Q:7, 9. Chicago.

American Hospital Association. *Coding Clinic for ICD-9-CM* 2009e, 2Q:7. Chicago.

American Hospital Association. *Coding Clinic for ICD-9-CM* 2006, 4Q:190. Chicago.

American Hospital Association. *Coding Clinic for ICD-9-CM* 2004, 3Q:4. Chicago.

American Hospital Association. *Coding Clinic for ICD-9-CM* 2000, 3Q:6 Chicago.

American Hospital Association. *Coding Clinic for ICD-9-CM* 1992, 2Q:15–16. Chicago.

American Hospital Association. *Coding Clinic for ICD-9-CM* 1986, March/April, 12. Chicago.

American Medical Association. 2010a. CPT *Current Procedural Terminology, Changes and Insider's View.* Chicago. AMA.

American Medical Association. 2010b. *CPT Current Procedural Terminology.* Professional Edition. Chicago. AMA.

Brodnik, M., C. McCain, M., Rinehart-Thompson, L., and R. Reynolds. 2009 *Fundamentals of Law for Health Informatics and Information Management,* Chicago: American Health Information Management Association.

Brown, F. 2009. *ICD-9-CM Coding Handbook with Answers.* Chicago: American Hospital Association.

Casto, A. and E. Layman. 2009. *Principles of Healthcare Reimbursement,* 2nd ed. Chicago: American Health Information Management Association.

Centers of Medicare and Medicaid. 2010a. National Correct Coding Initiative Edits http://www.cms.hhs.gov/NationalCorrectCodInitEd/.*

Centers of Medicare and Medicaid. 2010b. National Correct Coding Initiative, Medically Unlikely Edits http://www.cms.hhs.gov/NationalCorrectCodInitEd/08_MUE.asp#TopOfPage.

Centers for Medicare and Medicaid Services and the National Center for Health Statistics. 2010c. *ICD-9-CM Official Guidelines for Coding and Reporting.* http://www.cdc.gov/nchs/data/icd9/icdguide09.pdf.*

Centers of Medicare and Medicaid. 2010c. Nursing Home Quality Initiatives. http://www.cms.hhs.gov/NursingHomeQualityInits/25_NHQIMDS30.asp#TopOfPage.*

Centers of Medicare and Medicaid 2010d (February). http://www.cms.hhs.gov/MLNMattersArticles/downloads/MM6563.pdf.*

Centers of Medicare and Medicaid 2010e (February). http://www.cms.hhs.gov/ContractorLearningResources/downloads/JA6563.pdf.*

Department of Health and Human Services. 2003. Office of Inspector General, Medicare's National Correct Coding Initiative. 2003 (Sept.) OEI-03-02-00770.

Department of Health and Human Services, Centers for Disease Control and Prevention. 2010 http://www.cdc.gov/ncidod/dhqp/ar_kp.html.*

Dorland's Illustrated Medical Dictionary 30th **edition.** 2003. Philadelphia: Saunders.

Drugs.com. 2009 (November). http://www.drugs.com/protonix.html.*

Drugs.com. 2010a (April). http://www.drugs.com/cdi/retrovir.html.*

Drugs.com. 2010b (April). www.drugs.com/pdr/haldol.html.*

Gelzer, R. et al. 2008. AHIMA Copy Functionality Toolkit. http://www.ahima.org/infocenter/documents/copy_functionality_toolkit.pdf. Chicago: AHIMA.*

Hart, Anita C., Melinda S. Stegman, and Beth Ford (editors). 2009. *ICD-9-CM Professional 2010 for Hospitals—Volumes 1, 2, and 3,* Sixth Edition. Ingenix.

Hazelwood, A. and C. Venable. 2010. *ICD-9-CM Diagnostic Coding and Reimbursement for Physician Services*. Chicago: AHIMA.

Hirsch, R. 2006. Practice toolkit: medical record completion. *Journal of AHIMA* 77(1).

Johns, M.L. (ed). 2007. *Health Information Management Technology: An Applied Approach*. AHIMA. Chicago.

Joint Commission. (revised) 2009 (March). The Official Do Not Use List (April 2005). http://www.jointcommission.org/PatientSafety/DoNotUseList/ and http://www.jointcommission.org/PatientSafety/DoNotUseList/facts_dnu.htm.*

Kuehn, L. 2010. *Procedural Coding and Reimbursement for Physician Services: Applying Current Procedural Terminology and HCPCS*, Chicago: AHIMA.

LaTour, K. and S. Eichenwald Maki, eds. 2010. *Health Information Management: Concepts, Principles, and Practice*, 3rd edition., Chicago: AHIMA.

MacDonald, M. 2007. *Access 2007: The Missing Manual*. O'Reilly Media, Inc. Sebastopol, CA.

Merck Manuals Online Library. 2008a (April). www.merck.com/mmhe/sec04/ch042/ch042a.html?qt=pneumonia&alt=sh.*

Merck Manuals Online Library. 2008b (February). http://www.merck.com/mmhe/sec03/ch033/ch033c.html?qt=myocardial infarction&alt=sh#sec03-ch033-ch033c-933.*

Merck Manuals Online Library. 2008c (April) http://www.merck.com/mmhe/sec04/ch042/ch042e.html.*

Micheletti, J., A. Shlala, and J. Thomas. 2006. Documentation Rx: strategies for improving physician contribution to hospital records. *Journal of AHIMA* 77(2).

National Institute of Standards and Technology (NIST). 2006. *An Introduction to Computer Security: The NIST Handbook*. Special Publication 800-12. http://csrc.nist.gov/publications/nistpubs/800-12/.*

Odom-Wesley, B., D. Brown, and C. Meyers. 2009. *Documentation for Medical Records*, Chicago: American Health Information Management Association.

Pozgar, G.D. 2009. *Legal Essentials of Health Care Administration*. Sudbury, MA: Jones and Bartlett.

Russo, R. 2010. *Clinical Documentation Improvement: Achieving Excellence*. AHIMA: Chicago.

Schraffenberger, L.A. 2010. *Basic ICD-9-CM Coding*, Chicago: American Health Information Management Association.

Schraffenberger, L.A. 2008. Analysis of POA and hospital-acquired conditions data, part 1. *Journal of AHIMA* 79(6).

Servais, C. 2008. *The Legal Health Record.* AHIMA: Chicago.

Smith, G. 2010. *Basic Current Procedural Terminology and HCPCS Coding,* Chicago: AHIMA.

Thomason, M. and J. Dennis. 2008. *HIPAA by Example.* AHIMA: Chicago.

Links to URLs listed here can be found on the CD-ROM that accompanies this book.

Certified Coding Associate
Exam Preparation

Blank Answer Sheets

Printable blank answer sheets are also available
on the CD-ROM that accompanies this book.

Practice Answers

1. _____	41. _____	81. _____	121. _____	161. _____
2. _____	42. _____	82. _____	122. _____	162. _____
3. _____	43. _____	83. _____	123. _____	163. _____
4. _____	44. _____	84. _____	124. _____	164. _____
5. _____	45. _____	85. _____	125. _____	165. _____
6. _____	46. _____	86. _____	126. _____	166. _____
7. _____	47. _____	87. _____	127. _____	167. _____
8. _____	48. _____	88. _____	128. _____	168. _____
9. _____	49. _____	89. _____	129. _____	169. _____
10. _____	50. _____	90. _____	130. _____	170. _____
11. _____	51. _____	91. _____	131. _____	171. _____
12. _____	52. _____	92. _____	132. _____	172. _____
13. _____	53. _____	93. _____	133. _____	173. _____
14. _____	54. _____	94. _____	134. _____	174. _____
15. _____	55. _____	95. _____	135. _____	175. _____
16. _____	56. _____	96. _____	136. _____	176. _____
17. _____	57. _____	97. _____	137. _____	177. _____
18. _____	58. _____	98. _____	138. _____	178. _____
19. _____	59. _____	99. _____	139. _____	179. _____
20. _____	60. _____	100. _____	140. _____	180. _____
21. _____	61. _____	101. _____	141. _____	181. _____
22. _____	62. _____	102. _____	142. _____	182. _____
23. _____	63. _____	103. _____	143. _____	183. _____
24. _____	64. _____	104. _____	144. _____	184. _____
25. _____	65. _____	105. _____	145. _____	185. _____
26. _____	66. _____	106. _____	146. _____	186. _____
27. _____	67. _____	107. _____	147. _____	187. _____
28. _____	68. _____	108. _____	148. _____	188. _____
29. _____	69. _____	109. _____	149. _____	189. _____
30. _____	70. _____	110. _____	150. _____	190. _____
31. _____	71. _____	111. _____	151. _____	191. _____
32. _____	72. _____	112. _____	152. _____	192. _____
33. _____	73. _____	113. _____	153. _____	193. _____
34. _____	74. _____	114. _____	154. _____	194. _____
35. _____	75. _____	115. _____	155. _____	195. _____
36. _____	76. _____	116. _____	156. _____	196. _____
37. _____	77. _____	117. _____	157. _____	197. _____
38. _____	78. _____	118. _____	158. _____	198. _____
39. _____	79. _____	119. _____	159. _____	199. _____
40. _____	80. _____	120. _____	160. _____	200. _____

Practice Exam 1 Answers

1. _____ 41. _____ 81. _____
2. _____ 42. _____ 82. _____
3. _____ 43. _____ 83. _____
4. _____ 44. _____ 84. _____
5. _____ 45. _____ 85. _____
6. _____ 46. _____ 86. _____
7. _____ 47. _____ 87. _____
8. _____ 48. _____ 88. _____
9. _____ 49. _____ 89. _____
10. _____ 50. _____ 90. _____
11. _____ 51. _____ 91. _____
12. _____ 52. _____ 92. _____
13. _____ 53. _____ 93. _____
14. _____ 54. _____ 94. _____
15. _____ 55. _____ 95. _____
16. _____ 56. _____ 96. _____
17. _____ 57. _____ 97. _____
18. _____ 58. _____ 98. _____
19. _____ 59. _____ 99. _____
20. _____ 60. _____ 100. _____
21. _____ 61. _____
22. _____ 62. _____
23. _____ 63. _____
24. _____ 64. _____
25. _____ 65. _____
26. _____ 66. _____
27. _____ 67. _____
28. _____ 68. _____
29. _____ 69. _____
30. _____ 70. _____
31. _____ 71. _____
32. _____ 72. _____
33. _____ 73. _____
34. _____ 74. _____
35. _____ 75. _____
36. _____ 76. _____
37. _____ 77. _____
38. _____ 78. _____
39. _____ 79. _____
40. _____ 80. _____

Practice Exam 2 Answers

1. _____ 41. _____ 81. _____
2. _____ 42. _____ 82. _____
3. _____ 43. _____ 83. _____
4. _____ 44. _____ 84. _____
5. _____ 45. _____ 85. _____
6. _____ 46. _____ 86. _____
7. _____ 47. _____ 87. _____
8. _____ 48. _____ 88. _____
9. _____ 49. _____ 89. _____
10. _____ 50. _____ 90. _____
11. _____ 51. _____ 91. _____
12. _____ 52. _____ 92. _____
13. _____ 53. _____ 93. _____
14. _____ 54. _____ 94. _____
15. _____ 55. _____ 95. _____
16. _____ 56. _____ 96. _____
17. _____ 57. _____ 97. _____
18. _____ 58. _____ 98. _____
19. _____ 59. _____ 99. _____
20. _____ 60. _____ 100. _____
21. _____ 61. _____
22. _____ 62. _____
23. _____ 63. _____
24. _____ 64. _____
25. _____ 65. _____
26. _____ 66. _____
27. _____ 67. _____
28. _____ 68. _____
29. _____ 69. _____
30. _____ 70. _____
31. _____ 71. _____
32. _____ 72. _____
33. _____ 73. _____
34. _____ 74. _____
35. _____ 75. _____
36. _____ 76. _____
37. _____ 77. _____
38. _____ 78. _____
39. _____ 79. _____
40. _____ 80. _____